SLEEP APNEA - RECENT UPDATES

Edited by **Mayank G. Vats**

Sleep Apnea - Recent Updates
http://dx.doi.org/10.5772/62967
Edited by Mayank G. Vats

Contributors

Gurkan Rasit Rasit Bayar, Tamer Zerener, Rajiv Garg, Anand Srivastava, Jagadeesh H.N., Samson Assefa, Montserrat Diaz-Abad, Steven Scharf, Liselotte Sonnesen, José A. Vega, Teresa Cobo, Emilio Macias, Covadonga Alvarez, Juan Cobo, Felix Del Campo, Daniel Álvarez, Ana Cerezo-Hernández, Graciela López-Muñiz, Tania Álvaro-De Castro, Tomás Ruiz-Albi, Roberto Hornero

Published by InTech
Janeza Trdine 9, 51000 Rijeka, Croatia

Publishing Process Manager Romina Skomersic
Technical Editor SPi Global
Cover InTech Design team

First published April, 2017
Printed in Croatia
Legal deposit, Croatia: National and University Library in Zagreb

Additional hard copies can be obtained from orders@intechopen.com

Sleep Apnea - Recent Updates, Edited by Mayank G. Vats
p. cm.
Print ISBN 978-953-51-3055-0
Online ISBN 978-953-51-3056-7

For EU product safety concerns:
IN TECH d.o.o., Prolaz Marije Krucifikse Kozulić 3, 51000 Rijeka, Croatia,
info@intechopen.com or visit our website at intechopen.com.

Meet the editor

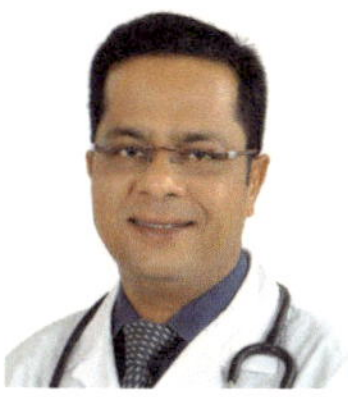

Dr. Mayank G. Vats is currently providing his services as the senior specialist in the Department of Pulmonary Medicine and Allergy and Sleep Medicine, Rashid Hospital, Dubai. His main area of research and clinical interest includes asthma, respiratory allergy, COPD, and sleep medicine. Dr. Vats completed his postgraduate education (MD) in Pulmonary Medicine; then, he did DNB in Respiratory Medicine and DNB in Critical Care medicine from the prestigious Escorts Heart Institute in New Delhi, India, and then served as a consultant pulmonologist, intensivist, and sleep physician at Escorts Heart Institute and Apollo Hospital, New Delhi, India, for more than 5 years. Previously, he provided his services as the specialist in the Department of Medicine and Chest Disease, Al Qassimi Hospital, Sharjah, UAE. Dr. Vats also got extensive training in sleep medicine by the American Academy of Sleep Medicine at LDS Hospital, Salt Lake City, Utah, USA, and at Cleveland Sleep Disorders Research Center. Dr. Vats got the membership of Royal College of Physicians and Surgeons of Glasgow, UK, and was elected as a fellow of the American College of Physicians (FACP) and fellow of the American College of Chest Physicians (FCCP). He is the European diplomat in respiratory medicine. Dr. Vats is the member in good standing of various medical professional societies, like ERS, ACCP, AASM, APSR, and ISCCM, to name a few. He has authored many peer-reviewed articles including original research, case reports, review articles, and chapters published in international books and journals and edited two books on respiratory medicine. He is presently also involved in many research projects, clinical trials, guideline projects in Gulf countries, and academic activities for the specialist doctors in UAE.

Contents

Preface

Sleep disorders are rampantly rising throughout the world and affect people of all ages, gender, and ethnicity. Inadequate sleep, poor in quantity and quality, and an excessive daytime sleepiness negatively affect daily activities of life. It's estimated that in the USA around 60–70 million people suffer from sleep disorder, and in developing countries sleep disease affects more than 200 million people. Considering the significant magnitude of sleep disorders, there is an increasing interest in sleep medicine among physicians, researchers, and the general public.

Sleep medicine is a relatively new specialty, still developing, although sleep has remained an important area of curiosity since the human civilization with emphasis on the physiologic and psychological basis and significance of sleep by many famous scientists.

Since then and especially in the past few years, sleep medicine is developing rapidly with more than 100 sleep disorders discovered till now. Despite that, sleep specialty is in neonatal stage especially in developing and underdeveloped countries. Sleep medicine is still evolving with an ongoing worldwide clinical research, training programs, and changes in the insurance policy disseminating more awareness in physicians and patients.

Sleep apnea is one of the most common sleep disorders, found in around 5–7% of the general population with high prevalence in the obese, elderly individuals but largely unrecognized and hence undiagnosed with untreated and life-threatening consequences.

In the last decade, new complex sleep disorders and its pathophysiology have been discovered, new treatments options (pharmacological and nonpharmacological) are available, and hence we planned a book on the recent developments on one of the most common sleep disorders, sleep apnea.

We have incorporated chapters from the eminent clinicians and authors around the globe to produce a state-of-the-art book with the target audience from internal medicine, pulmonary, sleep medicine, neurology, ENT, and psychiatry discipline.

With the blessings of the almighty God and my parents, this important task has been completed in a successful way.

I would like to convey special thanks to my wife Dr. Deepa Vats, who has special interest in pediatric sleep medicine, and my daughters Spraha Vats and Aadhya Vats for their constant and untiring support and encouragement.

Dr. Mayank G. Vats

Senior Specialist,

Pulmonologist, Intensivist, and Sleep Physician

Rashid Hospital and Dubai Hospital, Dubai, UAE

Chapter 1

Sleep Apnea – Recent Updates

Samson Z. Assefa, Montserrat Diaz-Abad and
Steven M. Scharf

Additional information is available at the end of the chapter

http://dx.doi.org/10.5772/66816

Abstract

Sleep apnea is highly prevalent and underdiagnosed. It is associated with multiple medical conditions including cardiac dysrhythmia, stroke, hypertension, diabetes and congestive heart failure. In the last few decades, advances in diagnosis and treatment of sleep apnea have been robust. In this review, we will emphasize primarily developments in the area of sleep apnea that occurred in the past 5 years. These include changes in the nomenclature of sleep apnea in the International Classification in Sleep Disorders (ICSD)-3, physiologic approach of treating sleep apnea, eligibility for CPAP (continuous positive airway pressure) treatment, home sleep testing (HST), sleep apnea in pregnancy, updates in oral device treatment and other emerging concepts on sleep apnea.

Keywords: sleep apnea, sleep apnea updates, obstructive sleep apnea, apnea, recent updates of sleep apnea

1. Introduction

Obstructive sleep apnea (OSA) is a prevalent condition associated with increased risk of developing hypertension, heart failure, type 2 diabetes, cardiac rhythm disturbances, stroke and increased all-cause mortality [1–7]. It is also associated with reduced quality of life and sleepiness. In the field of sleep disorders particularly diagnosis and treatment of sleep apnea continues to evolve. In this review article, we consider advances in our understanding of pathophysiology, diagnosis and treatment sleep apnea with emphasis on recent advances over the past 5 years.

Sleep disordered breathing (SDB) events are classified as *obstructive, central* or *mixed*. Furthermore, events are usually subdivided into *apneas* (complete or almost complete cessation of airflow), *hypopneas* (reduction of airflow by 30-90% associated with EEG arousals and/or 3-4 % oxygen desaturation) and *respiratory event-related arousals* (RERA—reduction of airflow by <30% associated with flow limitation and arousals on EEG) [8]. Obstructive events occur as a result of partial or complete obstruction of the upper airway at the level of the oro and/or nasopharynx with continuing respiratory efforts. Central events occur as a result of partial or complete cessation of efferent respiratory signals from the brainstem. Mixed events start out as central and evolve into obstructive events. Disordered breathing events (DBE) may be associated with reductions in oxygen saturation, sympathetic and parasympathetic surges and, in the case of obstructive events, large swings in intrathoracic pressure. Treatments for obstructive sleep apnea have classically included CPAP, certain types of upper airway surgery, dental orthotic or mandibular advancement devices, weight loss and positional therapy [9].

In the ensuing review, we discuss recent advances in the field including means of diagnosis and treatment in light of currently available literature.

2. Sleep-related breathing disorders nomenclature in ICSD-3

In the year of 2014, the American Academy of Sleep Medicine (AASM) released the 3rd edition of International Classification in Sleep Disorders (ICSD) [10]; this was an upgrade to the ICSD-2, 2011 edition. This shows progressive evolution of the nosology as knowledge and literature related to sleep disorders become more robust. There is a significant content change in the new edition, and one of them is within the sleep-related breathing disorders section. Treatment-central sleep apnea now appears as an isolated term to be used to describe central sleep apnea in the context of positive airway pressure treatment for obstructive sleep apnea. Other central sleep apneas like Cheyne-Stokes and substance induced are not classified in the same category. The other change in the SDB section is a separate diagnosis called sleep-related hypoxemia. This was under the same category of hypoventilation in the previous edition. In the ICSD-2, different categories based on the causes of the hypoxemia/hypoventilation that include medical and neurologic were listed separately. In ICSD-3, the cause of the hypoxemia/hypoventilation has to be diagnosed separately. Sleep-related hypoxemia diagnosis is assigned if a sleep study showed a sustained drop in SaO_2 but normal or not measured $PaCO_2$. In ICSD-3, obesity hypoventilation is also listed as a separate disorder due to its distinct clinical behavior. This requires a documentation of awake $PaCO_2$ >45 mm Hg. Refer to ICSD-3 for detailed review of the changes in all other sections [10].

3. Home sleep testing (HST)

OSA is prevalent and carries numerous physiologic and clinical consequences. The most recent prevalence estimates are that OSA is found in 33.9% of men and 17.4% of women [11]. These estimates are greater than previous ones, possibly due to increased sensitivity of detection, changes in definitions of types of "events," and/or increasing rates of obesity [11, 12]. Furthermore, as untreated sleep apnea is associated with a range of adverse consequences

[13], it has become clear that diagnostic testing needs to be convenient and available. Traditionally, in-laboratory attended polysomnography (PSG), in which sleep staging and cardiorespiratory variables are continuously recorded, has been the preferred method for diagnosing OSA. However, relatively high cost and growing wait times have provided the impetus for simplified portable unattended systems suitable for diagnosis of OSA outside the laboratory environment. In 1994 [14], AASM published a classification scheme grading the complexity of diagnostic sleep testing (see **Table 1**). Under this system, level 1 refers to commonly used in-laboratory attended PSG, level 2 refers to equally complex attended studies at home (rarely done) and levels 3 and 4 refer to unattended studies most commonly done at home, or out of the sleep laboratory. Since the original AASM classification system was published, technological advances have led to the availability of portable monitoring devices that may not neatly fit into the classification scheme. A revised system was presented in 2011 [15] similar to the 1994 system, but categorized portable devices according to the type of recording channel and the technology utilized. One of the primary issues is whether or not the device can adequately differentiate sleep from wakefulness and even stages of sleep. Many portable monitoring systems do not directly measure sleep using an EEG, but rather use derivative signals such as movement (actigraphy), pulse wave coupling or other derivative signals. For many systems, disease severity is more appropriately expressed as "respiratory disturbance index (RDI)" or "respiratory event index (REI)" (number of apneas/hypopneas per hour in bed) rather than the traditional apnea hypopnea index (apneas/hypopneas per hour of sleep) (AHI).

Level	Characteristics
1	Attended full PSG—the "gold standard" (EEG, sleep staging with four or more additional parameters, attended) CPT code: 95810 (Dx); 95811 (PAP, RAD); 95805 (MSLT/MWT)
2	Full PSG unattended/out of laboratory: as above—minimum 7 channels. HCPCS: G0398
3	Unattended, recording HR, O_2 saturation, respiratory airflow, respiratory effort; minimum of four channels, CPT: 95806; HCPCS: G0399
4	Unattended, HR, O_2 saturation, respiratory analysis; one or two channels, usually O_2 saturation or nasal airflow; CPT 95800 (includes estimated sleep time); 95801 (no sleep time); HCPCS G0400

Table 1. Levels of sleep testing (4).

A complete review of all home testing systems available is beyond the scope of this review. However, **Table 2** presents examples of several of the available simpler systems that have been validated. Both the AASM and the Canadian Sleep Society have published guidelines for use of portable monitors, most recently in 2010 [10]. These guidelines generally follow the highly selective study criteria outlined in validation studies. Portable monitoring devices are appropriate for patients with a high pretest probability of moderate-to-severe OSA (AHI of 15 or greater), but are not appropriate for routine screening in asymptomatic patients, or patients with concomitant medical or sleep disorders, such as central sleep apnea or periodic limb movement disorder. The Centers for Medicare and Medicaid Services (CMS) has approved coverage for PAP devices for patients diagnosed with OSA using portable monitoring [11].

System	Level	Principles/comments	References
Apnea risk evaluation system (ARES)[R]: SleepMed, Inc	3	Directly measures airflow, estimates respiratory effort from forehead vein, measures O_2 saturation and pulse rate. Approximates sleep time using lack of head movement	[6]
WatchPat[R] device: Itamar Medical Ltd	3*	Uses proprietary algorithm combined peripheral arterial tonometry, oximetry, heart rate, actigraphy to estimate sleep time and calculate respiratory disturbance index	[7]
Photoplethysmograph[R]: MorpheusOx; Widemed ltd.	3*	Measures O_2 saturation, pulse, peripheral arterial tone from optical volumetric signals. Proprietary algorithm detects sleep, respiration and disordered breathing events	[8]
ApneaStrip[R]: S.L.P. Ltd	3*	Simple device records airflow overnight and estimates sleep time	[9]

*Level claimed by manufacturer.

Table 2. Examples of portable home testing equipment (validation studies).

Many third party payers have followed CMS' lead; and in fact, many have instituted policies whereby portable sleep testing is required for all covered patients, with certain exceptions. Indeed in the highly selected patient populations studied for validation of portable testing, the correlation and even clinical outcomes are comparable between using portable diagnostic and in-laboratory testing [12–14]. However, as pointed out in an editorial by Collop [15], the issue is not the test *per se*, but how the test is utilized when it is "generalized." Most home sleep testing studies are done with highly selected patients (for the study quoted in Ref. [16], 272 patients were highly screened, 102 were randomized, approximately half to home testing). Furthermore, patients were evaluated by sleep experts, and scoring was done by well-trained and motivated technologists. Exclusions for significant medical, psychiatric and sleep disorders were rigidly carried out. However, in the "real world," as insurance carriers try to minimize costs, the experience is often that these conditions are not met. The decision to accept and indeed to "push for" home testing is often made on the basis of business and finance rather than patient benefit. While home or out of center sleep testing offers a number of advantages compared with in-laboratory PSG, there is no evidence that using this approach for all or the majority of patients is advantageous, even financially. The initial costs are generally less than those of in-laboratory testing. Furthermore, home testing offers a more rapid method of assessing the many patients with undiagnosed OSA who have limited access to, or who are reluctant to undergo, in-laboratory PSG. However, Chervin et al. [17] performed a careful cost utility analysis, comparing in-laboratory PSG, out of center testing and no testing (with treatment based on clinical characteristics). Their outcomes were based on costs per quality-adjusted life years over 5 years. These authors concluded that standard in-lab PSG provides greater quality-adjusted life years over 5 years than either out of center testing or no testing. Reuveni et al. [18] modeled costs of in-laboratory PSG versus out of center testing, accounting for the published technical failure rate of out of center testing, and the published European costs for PSG. They demonstrated that there was no long-term cost saving using out of center testing versus in-laboratory PSG.

Given that sleep apnea is under-diagnosed, another advantage of HST is diagnosing patients in a hospital setting and arranging follow-ups for complete evaluation in out-patient settings. Kauta et al. [19] evaluated 104 cardiac patients with SDB symptoms who are hospitalized for heart failure, arrhythmia and myocardial infarction. They performed type III portable sleep study, and 78% had SDB (AHI >5 events/h). Patients diagnosed with SDB were started with PAP treatment. At 30 days, adherence to PAP and 30-day readmission rate were assessed. None (0%) of patients (0/19) with adequate adherence, 30% of patients with partial adherence (6/20) and 29% of non-users (5/17) were readmitted or visited emergency room for cardiac issues ($p = 0.025$).

4. Effects of different definitions of DBEs on CPAP eligibility

Treatment with CPAP is known to significantly reduce the risk of important cardiovascular events and overall health care utilization [20, 21]. Thus, diagnosis and treatment of OSA would be expected to have a considerable beneficial impact on public health. Eligibility for CPAP treatment is usually based on disease severity, and this is usually expressed as the AHI. Of course, the number of events must perforce be based on the specific definitions of apneas, hypopneas and specified comorbid conditions. In 2012, the AASM adopted modified definitions of DBEs [8]. However, some insurance carriers including CMS continued to use the 2007 AASM definitions of DBEs [22]. The definitions of apneas between 2007 and 2012 have not changed [23], that is, a >90% reduction in airflow with continuing respiratory effort (for obstructive events). However, the 2012 AASM definition of hypopneas [8] calls for a 30–90% reduction in airflow associated with either a 3% reduction in O_2 saturation or a terminal arousal. The current CMS definition of hypopneas calls for the same reduction in airflow, but associated with a 4% reduction in O_2 saturation [23]. Further CMS defines the eligibility for CPAP treatment based on the AHI as follows: Patients are eligible for CPAP treatment for AHI ≥ 15, or if AHI is 5–14, only if the patient has a specified comorbidity, including hypertension, excessive sleepiness, impaired cognition, mood disorder, insomnia, ischemic heart disease, and history of stroke. Since CMS is often used by other insurance carriers as a model for designing their own treatment criteria, the differences in hypopnea definitions or in designation of treatment eligibility could have real significance.

Ho et al. [24] recently reviewed data on 6441 patients from the sleep heart health study and found, not surprisingly, that there was a discrepancy in the AHI depending on the definitions used for hypopneas, the discrepancy being greater at low AHIs than at high ones. Korotinsky et al. [25] recently compared AHI's calculated using both AASM (2012) and CMS definitions of hypopneas, as well as eligibility for CPAP treatment in a convenience sample of 112 consecutive patients studied in their sleep laboratory. Eighty-five patients were <65 years old and 27 were >65 years old (eligible for Medicare). They found the largest discrepancies in the younger patients, but a nonstatistically significant difference in the older patients. Furthermore, because of the presence of comorbidities in the older patients, there were no differences in eligibility for CPAP no matter which set of criteria were used. Thus, in younger patients, application of the stricter CMS criteria would have resulted in fewer patients being eligible for CPAP treatment, but not in the older patients. Thus, in the younger patients, application of the stricter CMS criteria for eligibility for CPAP treatment would have resulted in fewer patients with relatively mild (AHI, 5–14) OSA being treated with CPAP. The question as to whether there is a healthcare advantage for treatment of younger patients with mild disease is still unsettled with opinions on both sides of the question [25].

5. Toward a physiologic approach to treating OSA

Breathing involves a complex neurologic interaction of various types of inspiratory muscles. During inspiration, pressures down the airway are slightly negative, since air must move from atmospheric pressure (= 0) to alveoli (pressure slightly negative). Prior to activation of the diaphragm, there is the activation of upper airway/pharyngeal dilator muscles that prevent collapse of the upper airway during inspiration. Thus, the upper airway performs an important function during respiration, and if function is compromised, obstruction could result as in OSA [26, 27]. CPAP is one of the preferred treatments for moderate-to-severe OSA. However, since upper airway dilator stimulation is thought to be inadequate to maintain upper airway patency during sleep, especially during REM sleep when skeletal muscle tone is suppressed, the concept developed that electrical stimulation of upper airway dilator muscles during inspiration could help maintain airway patency. Thus, a number of systems have been developed whereby stimulation of a hypoglossal nerve through an implantable device, timed to the patient's normal inspiration could help to maintain airways patency and alleviate sleep apnea. This approach would be particularly useful in patients who cannot tolerate or refuse to tolerate CPAP or other treatments. Several clinical trials have been carried out on devices implanted subcutaneously that are, once activated, triggered by the patient's own inspiratory effort [27–33]. The largest of these [33], a multisite clinical trial of patients with moderate-to-severe OSA, surgically implanted a hypoglossal nerve stimulator in OSA patients who were CPAP intolerant or refused CPAP treatment. The primary outcome measures were AHI and the ODI4 (oxygen desaturation index—number of times per hour, O_2 saturation fell by at least 4%). Secondary outcomes included the Epworth Sleepiness Scale (ESS), the Functional Outcomes of Sleep Questionnaire and the percent of sleep time with oxygen saturation <90%. This single cohort included 126 patients. At the end of 1 year, the median AHI decreased from 29.3 per hour to 9.0 per hour with similar improvements in the ODI4. Quality of life (QOL) measures also improved at the end of 1 year. At the end of 1 year, 46 patients participated in a 1:1 randomized therapy withdrawal trial. In this phase, participants who had therapy withdrawn demonstrated return of disease severity compared with those in whom therapy was not withdrawn. **Table 3** lists appropriate criteria for therapy with a hypoglossal stimulator. Finally, it should be pointed out that implantation of a hypoglossal nerve stimulator is part of a comprehensive program that extends well beyond the surgical procedure. The complete details are beyond the scope of this review, but involve selection based on criteria presented in **Table 3**, endoscopic evaluation of pharyngeal collapse, training of patients and staff, and various stages of activation and titration of stimulation parameters.

http://dx.doi.org/10.5772/66816

Eligibility criteria
Age> 22 years
AHI (AASM) 20–65 events per hour sleep
Less than 25% of DBEs are central or mixed events
Body Mass Index (BMI)<32 Kg/m^2
Unable or unwilling to use CPAP (including non-compliers)
Based on criteria presented in Ref. [33].

Table 3. Criteria for consideration for hypoglossal nerve implantation.

6. Sleep apnea and telemedicine

As compared to the past few decades, there is a better sleep disorders recognition and understanding of the impacts. As a result, a number of patients who need integrated expertise of sleep medicine care have increased. However, there is a substantial shortage of sleep medicine specialists across the United States. AASM recognized telemedicine could be used as a tool to improve the specialist gap and deliver a cost-effective care while still maintaining high-quality care. The The American Telemedicine Association defines telemedicine as the use of medical information exchanged from one site to another via electronic communications to improve a patient's clinical health status. This includes e-mail, smart phones, wireless tools, two-way video and other forms of telecommunications technology [34].

Telemedicine has been implemented in the majority of the medical disciplines. In the early days, telemedicine was used in the field of sleep medicine mainly to promote and reinforce CPAP therapy adherence and showed mixed results. In other instances, transmission of sleep studies by non-specialist to a sleep specialist for review has been used [35]. Taylor et al. [36] randomly grouped patients to usual care and telemedicine-based adherence for CPAP. Usual care patients visited practitioners in clinics and patients on telemedicine group had computer-based monitoring device that did not include video conferencing. Participants are contacted either by phone or by computer-based system. The study found no significant difference between the two groups. Other limited telemedicine application was doing sleep studies and diagnosing sleep disorders. Mendelson et al. [37] in 2014 randomized a total of 107 hypertensive patients to CPAP care (n = 53) and CPAP care with a telemedicine intervention (n = 54). Patients assigned to telemedicine uploaded blood pressure (BP) measurement, CPAP adherence, sleepiness and quality of life data and in return on regular bases they received recommendations. The main outcome was home self-measurement of BP improvement. Telemedicine-supported CPAP users did not improve BP and cardiovascular risk in high-risk OSA patients.

In 2008, the Milwaukee Veterans Administration Medical Center evaluated the application of telemedicine in sleep medicine [38]. Based on electronic consult eligibility for portable study, patients were assessed and sleep study orders were placed by sleep specialists. The need for in-person assessment was also evaluated, and appointments were scheduled. CPAP was ordered for confirmed sleep apnea. Baig et al. [38] retrospectively assessed the 5-year trend in accessibility to and receipt of care after the program was implemented. They found that, in spite of increased volume of services, the interval between sleep consult and PAP prescription decreased from >60 days to <7 days. However, there was no change in clinic wait time of >60 days.

In the past decade, the use of tele-sleep medicine has been expanded to include patient's sleep evaluation. Before AASM came up with recommendation on telemedicine for sleep medicine, there were studies that supported telemedicine could be used for complete evaluation of sleep medicine patients. A pilot study by Spaulding et al. [39] showed the application of telemedicine that included video conferencing. The group established tele-heath service in a rural area of Kansas after training nurses and Registered Polysomnography Technologists (RPSGT) on how to use the videoconferencing webcam and intraoral camera for examining severity of airway narrowing. There were 18 new patients visits and four follow-ups. They reported that telemedicine was effective for physician-patient interaction and visualizing the upper airway. The only problem was nurses had to be trained to present patients and use the video cam and oral camera.

The AASM published a position paper in 2015 [40] that telemedicine can be used to improve access to sleep medicine services provided by board-certified sleep medicine specialist and improve communications with other specialties. Telemedicine applications can be broadly categorized into two: synchronous and asynchronous interactions. Synchronous is a live, real-time, bidirectional, audio-video conferencing provider-patient interaction who are distant apart. Tele-stethoscope and mobile cameras can be used for physical exam that is done in the presence of a presenter who usually is a trained nurse practitioner, physician assistant, respiratory therapist, RPSGT or medical office assistant. The patient presenter gives a clinical support and assistance with physical exam. Asynchronous evaluation uses multiple models and involves the encounters occur at different times and are communicated one directionally between patients and providers electronically. AASM recommended providers to adopt technical requirements from the American Telemedicine Guidelines [40]. AASM believes if the technical, organizational and healthcare professional requirements are met, synchronous encounters could function as live office visits.

In January 2016, the AASM officially launched AASM SleepTM. This is a telemedicine platform designed for the sleep medicine field. Some centers have implemented telemedicine. Issues that need further clarification while implementing telemedicine include cost uncertainties, reimbursement structure and licensing rules. Currently, expansion of telemedicine to all sleep disorders has its own restrictions and providers should refer to their local standard for the technical and organizational requirements.

7. Sleep apnea and pregnancy

7.1. Screening OSA during pregnancy

In general, sleep disturbances are highly prevalent during pregnancy including SDB. Self-reported snoring is common with a prevalence of 14–41% as compared with 4–17% in non-pregnant women [41–46]. Recognition of sleep apnea in pregnant women in particular is difficult because pregnancy is dynamic process and multiple studies at different time points during pregnancy may not be feasible. In 2015, there were two articles that tried to assess the screening tools for sleep apnea in pregnancy. Lockhart et al. [47] assessed 218 third trimester pregnancies of which 12% had sleep apnea diagnosed using portable home sleep testing. In this study STOP, STOP BANG, Berlin, American Society of Anesthesiologist Checklist and ESS were not successful in detecting sleep apnea. However, some of the elements such as BMI, neck circumference, diagnosis of hypertension (HTN) and falling asleep while talking to others where more predictive based on univariate and multivariate analysis. Tantrakul et al. [48] evaluated Berlin and STOP BANG questionnaires to detect OSA across trimesters of high-risk pregnancy. They consisted of n = 72 (first trimester n = 23, second trimester n = 24 and third trimester n = 25), and with prevalence of OSA by trimester from first to third was 30.4%, 33.3% and 32.0%, respectively. Overall, predictive values of Berlin and STOP BANG were fair (AUC 0.72 for Berlin, P = 0.003, 0.75 for STOP BANG, P = 0.0001). The predictive values performed poorer during the first trimester. Multivariant analyses showed pre-pregnancy BMI, snore frequently and weight gain/BMI were significantly associated with OSA in first, second and third trimesters, respectively. Izci et al. [46] demonstrated third trimester pregnant females have smaller mean pharyngeal areas when compared with postpartum in supine, lateral and seated positions with a mean difference of 0.20 (95% CI 0.06–0.35), 0.26 (95% CI 0.12–0.39) and 0.18 (95% CI 0.02–0.32), respectively.

7.2. OSA and perinatal outcomes

Repeated upper airway resistance and/or obstruction during sleep due to DBEs that causes chronic intermittent hypoxia, hypercarbia and sleep disruptions is believed to be a culprit for higher incidence of negative perinatal outcomes. However, studies have shown conflicting results. Tauman et al. [49] recruited 122 pregnant women with habitual snoring and 39% had SDB. In those pregnant women who snored had increased markers of fetal distress, which are circulating nucleated RBC, EPO and IL-6. However, there was no difference in neonatal outcome. Trudell et al. [50] conducted a study with the aim to develop a tool for airway assessment to predict adverse pregnancy outcomes. They hypothesized that higher Mallampati score (MS) is associated with adverse perinatal outcomes. Outcomes were compared between low MS and high MS in a total of 1823 term births. No significant difference was found in the risk of small for gestational age (SGA) [adjusted odds ratio 0.9 (95% CI 0.6–1.2), preeclampsia adjusted odds ratio 1.2 (95% CI 0.8–1.9) or neonatal acedemia 0.8 (95% CI 0.3–2)]. In recent population-based retrospective study (n = 636,227), Bin et al. [51] found that OSA was significantly associated with HTN, planned delivery, preterm birth, 5-min Apgar <7, admission to neonatal ICU/special care nursery and large for gestational age infant but was not associated with gestational diabetes, Cesarean section, perinatal death or SGA.

Trauman et al. [52] prospectively studied 74 pregnant women (24% with OSA) and full-term infants for general movements and neurodevelopment at 48 h, 8–11 weeks, 14–16 weeks and at 12 months. Infant developmental inventory and infant brief questioner were administered. At 12 months, 64% of infants born to SDB mothers showed low social developmental score as compared to 25% of infants born to controls (P = 0.36, odds ratio 16.7). In neonatal and infant neuromotor development, there was no difference between infants born to SBD mother or controls. Another study that failed to show negative outcome was by Bassan et al. [53]. The group studied 44 women (25% had SDB) with full-term infants showed that there was no difference in birthweight, gestational age, 5-min APGAR score and neurological exam score between infants born to SDB and non-SDB mothers.

Ravishankar et al. [54] studied the effect of SDB on histopathology and immune-histochemical markers of placental perfusion and hypoxia. The placentas of women with OSA (n = 23), habitual snoring (n = 78) and non-snorers (n = 47) were accessed. Fetal normoblastemia was prevalent in OSA as compared to snorers and controls (56.5%, 34.6%, and 6.4% respectively). Increased tissue hypoxia marker, carbonic anhydrase IX immunoreactivity, was demonstrated in OSA pregnant women as compare to non-snorers and controls (81.5%, 91.3% and 57.5%, respectively). Uteroplacental and reperfusion score were similar in all groups.

Further studies in the future are warranted to assess the effect of SDB on perinatal and neonatal outcome.

8. Update on oral appliance therapy

In 2015, the AASM published an update of clinical practice guidelines of treatment for OSA and snoring with oral appliance therapy [55]. The new guidelines continued to recommend oral appliance therapy and gave increased focus on patient preference. An oral appliance can now be considered for all levels of OSA severity (mild, moderate and severe), if the patient fails or refuses CPAP, or even if they simply prefer an oral appliance to CPAP.

Subjective adherence with oral appliance therapy is better overall than objective adherence with CPAP in adult patients with OSA. CPAP is superior to oral appliance therapy in improving the AHI and lowering the arousal index and the ODI, but the new guidelines suggest that the overall therapeutic effectiveness of oral appliances may be comparable with CPAP because of the significant difference in adherence rates.

These new guidelines recommend that sleep physicians prescribe oral appliances for patients who request treatment of primary snoring. When prescribed for OSA patient, it suggests that a qualified dentist use a custom, titratable appliance. It also recommends that sleep physicians consider prescription of oral appliances for adult patients with OSA who are intolerant of CPAP therapy or prefer alternate therapy. Qualified dentists should provide oversight of oral appliance therapy in OSA patients, and sleep physicians should conduct follow-up sleep testing to improve or confirm treatment efficacy.

Studies have demonstrated efficacy of oral appliance therapy comparable to CPAP in selected patients [56, 57]. While oral appliances help to decrease AHI/RDI/REI across all severity levels, there are few reported factors that consistently predict improvement in OSA using oral appliances. A number of possible predictors have been examined. Among these are changes in pharyngeal geometry under drug-induced sleep endoscopy (DISE) [58] and nasoendoscopy to assess velopharynx/oro/hypopharyngeal geometry [59]. In the study of Gjerde [57], low oxygen levels carried a high predictive value for failure with oral appliance therapy.

9. Update on PAP devices

Many types of PAP devices are used to treat the whole spectrum of SDB including CPAP, autotitrating CPAP (APAP), bilevel PAP, autotitrating bilevel PAP, volume-assured pressure support and adaptive servoventilation. CPAP and APAP are most commonly used, whereas the other modes are reserved for patients needing respiratory assist. For CPAP and APAP, data collection systems can track compliance, pressure, leak and efficacy. Refer to Johnson et al. [60] for a comprehensive review of the technological aspects of PAP devices in general with its algorithms, including event detection, sampling rates, cycling, targets, rate and pressure adjustments as well as suggested settings.

APAP has been shown to be an effective means to determine therapeutic CPAP levels. The question remains as to whether APAP is suitable for long-term treatment of patients with OSA. In the past 5 years, at least three different meta-analyses [61–63] have been performed comparing the efficacy of CPAP to APAP and demonstrating similar effectiveness. These three studies have found that APAP and CPAP produce comparable reductions in AHI, decreased sleepiness, comparable long-term compliance and improvements in sleep architecture. Because the treatment effects are similar between APAP and CPAP, the therapy of choice may depend on other factors such as patient preference, specific reasons for non-compliance and cost [62].

Although CPAP and APAP appear comparable, other investigators have looked at the use of alternative PAP modalities presumed to be more comfortable for therapy in OSA patients with the hopes of leading to improved compliance. These have included auto-bi-level pressure relief-positive airway pressure (ABPR-PAP). Four studies [64–67] showed similar improvements in symptoms using an auto-bi-level mode and CPAP. Compliance was generally better with the auto-bi-level modes than CPAP, even in CPAP patients selected for poor compliance [65, 67].

10. Emerging concepts

Over the past 5 years, there continues to be advancement in understanding of all aspects of OSA. Major categories have been covered in other areas of this review. Below is a selected group of topics with new emerging points of view that deserve increased focus in the future.

10.1. Interventions to improve CPAP compliance

CPAP is not accepted by many users. Educational, supportive and behavioral interventions may help people with OSA recognize the need for regular and continued use of CPAP. An updated review on the effect of these intervention modalities was performed in 2014. Thirty randomized controlled studies (2047 participants) were included [68]. Low-to-moderate quality evidence showed that all three types of interventions led to increased machine usage in CPAP-naive patients with moderate-to-severe OSA. Compared with usual care, supportive ongoing interventions increased CPAP use by 50 min per night and increased the number of patients who used CPAP for longer than 4 hours per night from 59% to 75%. Educational interventions increased CPAP use by 35 min per night and increased the number of patients who used CPAP for longer than 4 h per night from 57% to 70%. Behavioral therapy led to an improvement in CPAP use of 1.44 h per night and increased the number of patients who used CPAP for longer than four hours per night from 28% to 47%.

10.2. More focus on the relationship between smoking and OSA

It has been suspected for some time that smoking and OSA adversely affect each other, leading to increased comorbidity; however, this is still a matter of debate. There seems to be a synergistic effect between smoking and OSA, which may lead to increase in cardiovascular morbidity [69]. However, the evidence is less than conclusive. Cigarette smoking may increase the severity of OSA through alterations in sleep architecture, upper airway neuromuscular function, arousal mechanisms and upper airway inflammation. And untreated OSA may be associated with smoking addiction. The effect of smoking cessation on OSA remains to be determined. Future studies are needed in order to establish the strength of the association of both conditions [70].

11. Patient-specific therapy and customization of therapy

11.1. Focus on pathophysiology

There has been an increased focus on the importance of pathophysiological factor identification for customized therapy in OSA patients and more investigation of different group phenotypes or individual characteristics to personalize OSA therapy. Differentiated OSA phenotypes have been proposed: a small pharyngeal airway with a low resistance to collapse (increased critical closing pressure), an inadequate response of pharyngeal dilator muscles (wakefulness drive to breathe), an unstable ventilator responsiveness to hypercapnia (high loop gain) and an increased propensity to wake related to upper airway obstruction (low arousal threshold) [71]. If an accurate pathophysiological pattern for each OSA patient can be identified, customized—and presumably more effective—therapy would potentially be feasible [71].

A large cohort of 1249 patients (age 47 years; AHI 18.9/h; BMI 27.2 ± 3.7 kg/m^2) underwent PSG and DISE to determine upper airway (UA) collapse patterns [72]. Palatal collapse was the most frequent (81%). Multilevel collapse was noted in 68.2% of patients; the most frequent multilevel pattern was a combination of palatal and tongue base collapse (25.5%). The prevalence of complete collapse, multilevel collapse and hypopharyngeal collapse increased with increasing severity of obstructive sleep apnea (OSA). Multilevel and complete collapses were more prevalent in obese patients and in those with more severe OSA. Both higher BMI and AHI values were associated with a higher probability of complete concentric palatal collapse. However, UA collapse patterns during DISE cannot be fully explained by selected baseline polysomnographic and anthropometric characteristics.

Age may play a significant role. A study in which 10 young (20–40 year) and old (60 year and older) patients with OSA matched by BMI and sex suggested that airway anatomy/collapsibility plays a relatively greater pathogenic role in older adults whereas sensitive ventilatory control system is more prominent trait in younger adults [73].

11.2. Focus on mild OSA

There remains to be a debate about how significant is the effect of mild OSA on adverse health outcomes, to the point that unless not accompanied by specific medical conditions or symptoms, insurers will not cover therapy. The American Thoracic Society in 2016 published a research statement hoping to find answers to this lingering question [74]. The specific goals of this statement were to appraise the evidence regarding whether long-term adverse neurocognitive and cardiovascular outcomes are attributable to mild OSA and evaluate whether or not treatment of mild OSA is effective at preventing or reducing these adverse outcomes.

Unfortunately, studies were incongruent in their definitions of mild OSA, and data were inconsistent regarding the relationship between mild OSA and daytime sleepiness. It was concluded that treatment of mild OSA may improve sleepiness in patients who are sleepy at baseline and improve quality of life. There was limited or inconsistent evidence pertaining to the impact of therapy of mild OSA on other adverse outcomes.

11.3. More focus on perioperative care of OSA patients

The Society of Anesthesia and Sleep Medicine published in 2016 guidelines on preoperative screening and assessment of OSA patients [75]. This guideline emphasizes again the increased risks of perioperative complications in patients with OSA and recommended that practice groups consider making OSA screening a standard part pre-anesthetic evaluation. It did not go as far as recommending cancelling or delaying surgery to diagnose OSA unless there is evidence of an associated significant or uncontrolled systemic disease or additional problems with ventilation or gas exchange. The use of PAP therapy in previously undiagnosed, but suspected OSA patients should be considered case by case. Continued use of PAP therapy at previously prescribed settings in OSA is recommended during periods of sleep while hospitalized, both preoperatively and postoperatively. These guidelines strongly recommended for protocols for known or suspected OSA to be developed by individual institutions taking into account the patients' conditions, extent of interventions and available resources.

11.4. More focus on commercial motor vehicle OSA screening and treatment

A recommendation overview of commercial motor vehicle OSA screening and treatment was published in 2016. This document goes over prior recommendations and details the small differences present in other statements regarding this topic. There is a need for federal regulations to clarify the issue. Among the recommendations by the authors are the following [76]:

Out of service evaluation is recommended when admitted sleepiness while driving, motor vehicle collision attributable to falling asleep, ESS score >10, and OSA without objective documentation of sufficient therapy efficacy and/or adherence for OSA testing. PSG is preferred diagnostic test; however, HST may be a reasonable alternative in selected patients based on the sleep specialist assessment.

AHI, RDI or REI >20/h are recommended to have treatment. PAP therapy is generally the most expeditious treatment available. Surgical evaluation may be considered based on comprehensive assessment findings. Weight loss is recommended as adjunct. AHI, RDI or REI ≥5/h with sleepiness or sleepiness-related accident should be counseled to initiate treatment for OSA.

Documentation of efficacy of therapy is recommended. PAP therapy usage below published minimum recommendations (≥4 h for ≥70% of nights) could result in removal from service by the certified medical examiner. PAP therapy adherence should be objectively monitored by a sleep specialist assessing therapy adherence and efficacy. Printed reports of therapy adherence data should be made available to the certified medical examiner.

Author details

Samson Z. Assefa*, Monteserrat Diaz-Abad and Steven M. Scharf

*Address all correspondence to: sassefa1@medicine.umaryland.edu

University of Maryland, Baltimore, USA

References

[1] Fein AS, Shvilkin A, Shah D, Haffajee CI, Das S, Kumar K, et al. Treatment of obstructive sleep apnea reduces the risk of atrial fibrillation recurrence after catheter ablation. J Am Coll Cardiol 2013 Jul 23;62(4):300–305.

[2] Foster GD, Sanders MH, Millman R, Zammit G, Borradaile KE, Newman AB, et al. Obstructive sleep apnea among obese patients with type 2 diabetes. Diabetes Care 2009 Jun;32(6):1017–1019.

[3] Gottlieb DJ, Yenokyan G, Newman AB, O'Connor GT, Punjabi NM, Quan SF, et al. Prospective study of obstructive sleep apnea and incident coronary heart disease and heart failure: the sleep heart health study. Circulation 2010 Jul 27;122(4):352–360.

[4] O'Connor GT, Caffo B, Newman AB, Quan SF, Rapoport DM, Redline S, et al. Prospective study of sleep-disordered breathing and hypertension: the Sleep Heart Health Study. Am J Respir Crit Care Med 2009 Jun 15;179(12):1159–1164.

[5] Punjabi NM, Caffo BS, Goodwin JL, Gottlieb DJ, Newman AB, O'Connor GT, et al. Sleep-disordered breathing and mortality: a prospective cohort study. PLoS Med 2009 Aug;6(8):e1000132.

[6] Punjabi NM, Shahar E, Redline S, Gottlieb DJ, Givelber R, Resnick HE, et al. Sleep-disordered breathing, glucose intolerance, and insulin resistance: the Sleep Heart Health Study. Am J Epidemiol 2004 Sep 15;160(6):521–530.

[7] Redline S, Yenokyan G, Gottlieb DJ, Shahar E, O'Connor GT, Resnick HE, et al. Obstructive sleep apnea-hypopnea and incident stroke: the sleep heart health study. Am J Respir Crit Care Med 2010 Jul 15;182(2):269–277.

[8] Berry RB, Brooks R, Gamaldo CE, et al. for the American Academy of Sleep Medicine. The AASM Manual for the Scoring of Sleep and Associated Events: Rules, Terminology and Technical Specifications, Version 2.2, www.aasmnet.org, American Academy of Sleep Medicine, Darien, IL 2015. http://www.aasmnet.org/scoringmanual/v2.2.0/html/index.html

[9] Epstein LJ, Kristo D, Strollo PJ,Jr, Friedman N, Malhotra A, Patil SP, et al. Clinical guideline for the evaluation, management and long-term care of obstructive sleep apnea in adults. J Clin Sleep Med 2009 Jun 15;5(3):263–276.

[10] American Academy of Sleep Medicine. International Classification of Sleep Disorders, 3rd ed. American Academy of Sleep Medicine, Darien, IL 2014.

[11] Peppard PE, Young T, Barnet JH, Palta M, Hagen EW, Hla KM. Increased prevalence of sleep-disordered breathing in adults. Am J Epidemiol 2013 May 1;177(9):1006–1014.

[12] Heinzer R, Vat S, Marques-Vidal P, Marti-Soler H, Andries D, Tobback N, et al. Prevalence of sleep-disordered breathing in the general population: the HypnoLaus study. Lancet Respir Med 2015 Apr;3(4):310–318.

[13] Greenberg H, Lakticova V, Scharf SM. Obstructive sleep apnea: clinical features, evaluation and principles of management. In: Kryger M, Roth T, Dement WC (eds) Principles and Practices of Sleep Medicine, 6th ed. pp. 1110–1124; Elsevier, Philadelphia, PA 2016.

[14] Ferber R, Millman R, Coppola M, Fleetham J, Murray CF, Iber C, et al. Portable recording in the assessment of obstructive sleep apnea. ASDA standards of practice. Sleep 1994 Jun;17(4):378–392.

[15] Collop NA, Tracy SL, Kapur V, et al. Obstructive sleep apnea devices for out-of-center (OOC) testing: technology evaluation. J Clin Sleep Med 2011;7(5):531–548.

[16] Skomro RP, Gjevre J, Reid J, et al. Outcomes of home-based diagnosis and treatment of obstructive sleep apnea. Chest 2010;138 (2):257–263.

[17] Chervin RD, Murman DL, Malow BA, et al. Cost-utility of three approaches to the diagnosis of sleep apnea: polysomnography, home testing, and empirical therapy. Ann Intern Med 1999;130(6):496–505.

[18] Reuveni H, Schweitzer E, Tarasiuk A. A cost-effectiveness analysis of alternative at-home or in-laboratory technologies for the diagnosis of obstructive sleep apnea syndrome. Med Decis Making 2001;21(6):451–458.

[19] Kauta SR, Keenan BT, Goldberg L, Schwab RJ. Diagnosis and treatment of sleep disordered breathing in hospitalized cardiac patients: a reduction in 30-day hospital readmission rates. J Clin Sleep Med 2014 Oct 15;10(10):1051–1059.

[20] Marin JM, Carrizo SJ, Vicente E, Agusti AG. Long-term cardiovascular outcomes in men with obstructive sleep apnoea/hypopnoea with or without treatment with continuous positive airway pressure: an observational study. Lancet 2005;365:1046–1053.

[21] Otake K, Delaive K, Walld R, Manfreda J, Kryger MH. Cardiovascular medication use in patients with undiagnosed obstructive sleep apnoea. Thorax 2002;57:417–422.

[22] Iber C, Ancoli–Israel S, Chesson AL Jr, Quan SF. The AASM manual for the scoring of sleep and associated events: rules, terminology and technical specifications, 1st edn. American Academy of Sleep Medicine, Westchester, IL 2007

[23] Centers for Medicare and Medicaid Services (2001). Decision memo for continuous positive airway pressure (CPAP) therapy for obstructive sleep apnea (OSA) (CAG-00093 N). Available online at http://www.cms.gov/medicare-coverage-database/details/ncadecision-memo.aspx?NCAId = 19&fromdb = true.

[24] Ho V, Crainiceanu CM, Punjabi NM, Redline S, Gottlieb DJ. Calibration model for apnea-hypopnea indices: impact of alternative criteria for hypopneas. Sleep 2015;38:1887–1892.

[25] Korotinsky A, Assefa SZ, Diaz-Abad M, et al. Comparison of American Academy of Sleep Medicine (AASM) versus Center for Medicare and Medicaid Services (CMS) polysomnography (PSG) scoring rules on AHI and eligibility for continuous positive airway pressure (CPAP) treatment. Sleep Breath. 2016 Dec;20(4):1169–``1174.

[26] Pierce RJ, Worsnop CJ. Upper airway function and dysfunction in respiration. Clin Exp Pharm Phys 1999;26:1–10.

[27] Eckert DJ, Malholtra A, Lo UL, et al. The influence of obstructive sleep apnea and gender on genioglossus activity during rapid eye movement sleep. Chest 2009 April;135(4). doi:10.1378/chest.08–2292.

[28] Van de Heyning PH, Badr MS, Baskin JZ, et al. Implanted upper airway stimulation device for obstructive sleep apnea. Laryngoscope. 2012;122(7):1626–1633.

[29] Schwartz AR, Bennett ML, Smith PL, et al. Therapeutic electrical stimulation of the hypoglossal nerve in obstructive sleep apnea. Arch Otolaryngol Head Neck Surg 2001;127(10):1016–1023.

[30] Eastwood PR, Barnes M, Walsh JH, et al. Treating obstructive sleep apnea with hypoglossal nerve stimulation). Sleep 2011;34(11):1479–1486.

[31] Kent DT, Lee JJ, Strollo PJ Jr, Soose RJ. Upper Airway Stimulation for OSA: Early Adherence and Outcome Results of One Center. Otolaryngol Head Neck Surg. 2016 Jul;155(1):188–93.

[32] Safiruddin F, Vanderveken OM, de Vries N, et al. Effect of upper airway stimulation for obstructive sleep apnoea on airway dimension. Eur Respir J 2015;45(1):129–138.

[33] Strollo PJ Jr, Soose RJ, Maurer JT, et al. Upper airway stimulation for obstructive sleep apnea. NEJM 2014;370:139–149.

[34] American Telemedicine Association. http://www.americantelemed.org/about-telemedicine/what-is-telemedicine#.V9L_C_krLmg

[35] Boehning N, Blau A, Kujumdshieva B, Staubitz A, Boehning W. Preliminary results from a telemedicine referral network for early diagnosis of sleep apnoea in sleep laboratories. J Telemed Telecare 2009;15(4):203–207.

[36] Taylor Y, Eliasson A, Andrada T, Kristo D, Howard R. The role of telemedicine in CPAP compliance for patients with obstructive sleep apnea syndrome. Sleep Breath 2006 Sep;10(3):132–138.

[37] Mendelson M, Vivodtzev I, Tamisier R, Laplaud D, Dias-Domingos S, Baguet JP, et al. CPAP treatment supported by telemedicine does not improve blood pressure in high cardiovascular risk OSA patients: a randomized, controlled trial. Sleep 2014 Nov 1;37(11):1863–1870.

[38] Baig MM, Antonescu-Turcu A, Ratarasarn K. Impact of sleep telemedicine protocol in management of sleep apnea: a 5-year VA experience. Telemed J E Health 2016 May;22(5):458–462.

[39] Spaulding R, Stevens D, Velasquez SE. Experience with telehealth for sleep monitoring and sleep laboratory management. J Telemed Telecare 2011;17(7):346–349.

[40] Singh J, Badr MS, Diebert W, Epstein L, Hwang D, Karres V, et al. American Academy of Sleep Medicine (AASM) position paper for the use of telemedicine for the diagnosis and treatment of sleep disorders. J Clin Sleep Med 2015 Oct 15;11(10):1187–1198.

[41] Loube DI. Self-reported snoring in pregnancy. Association with fetal outcome. Chest 1996;109:885–889.

[42] Franklin KA. Snoring, pregnancy-induced hypertension and growth retardation of the fetus. Chest 2000;117:137–141.

[43] Pien GW, Schwab RJ. Sleep disorders during pregnancy. Sleep 2004;27:1405–1417.

[44] Leung PL, Hui DSC, Leung TN, Yuen PM, Lau TK. Sleep disturbances in Chinese pregnant women. BJOG 2005;112:1568–1571.

[45] Mindell JA, Cook RA, Nikolovski J. Sleep patterns and sleep disturbances across pregnancy. Sleep Med 2015 Apr;16(4):483–488.

[46] Izci B, Vennelle M, Liston WA, Dundas KC, Calder AA, Douglas NJ. Sleep-disordered breathing and upper airway size in pregnancy and post-partum. Eur Respir J 2006 Feb;27(2):321–327.

[47] Lockhart EM, Ben Abdallah A, Tuuli MG, Leighton BL. Obstructive sleep apnea in pregnancy: assessment of current screening tools. Obstet Gynecol 2015 Jul;126(1):93–102.

[48] Tantrakul V, Sirijanchune P, Panburana P, Pengjam J, Suwansathit W, Boonsarngsuk V, et al. Screening of obstructive sleep apnea during pregnancy: differences in predictive values of questionnaires across trimesters. J Clin Sleep Med 2015 Jan 15;11(2):157–163.

[49] Tauman R, Many A, Deutsch V, Arvas S, Ascher-Landsberg J, Greenfeld M, et al. Maternal snoring during pregnancy is associated with enhanced fetal erythropoiesis—a preliminary study. Sleep Med 2011 May;12(5):518–522.

[50] Trudell AS, Louis JM, Tuuli MG, Caughey AB, Odibo AO, Cahill AG. Use of a simple clinical tool for airway assessment to predict adverse pregnancy outcomes. Am J Perinatol 2015 Feb;32(3):257–262.

[51] Bin YS, Cistulli PA, Ford JB. Population-Based Study of Sleep Apnea in Pregnancy and Maternal and Infant Outcomes. J Clin Sleep Med. 2016 Jun 15;12(6):871–7.

[52] Tauman R, Zuk L, Uliel-Sibony S, Ascher-Landsberg J, Katsav S, Farber M, et al. The effect of maternal sleep-disordered breathing on the infant's neurodevelopment. Am J Obstet Gynecol 2015 May;212(5):656.e1–656.e7.

[53] Bassan H, Uliel-Sibony S, Katsav S, Farber M, Tauman R. Maternal sleep disordered breathing and neonatal outcome. Isr Med Assoc J 2016 Jan;18(1):45–48.

[54] Ravishankar S, Bourjeily G, Lambert-Messerlian G, He M, De Paepe ME, Gundogan F. Evidence of placental hypoxia in maternal sleep disordered breathing. Pediatr Dev Pathol 2015 Sep-Oct;18(5):380–386.

[55] Ramar K, Dort LC, Katz SG, Lettieri CJ, Harrod CG, Thomas SM, et al. Clinical practice guideline for the treatment of obstructive sleep apnea and snoring with oral appliance therapy: an update for 2015. J Clin Sleep Med 2015 Jul 15;11(7):773–827.

[56] Takaesu Y, Tsuiki S, Kobayashi M, Komada Y, Nakayama H, Inoue Y. Mandibular advancement device as a comparable treatment to nasal continuous positive airway pressure for positional obstructive sleep apnea. J Clin Sleep Med 2016 Aug 15;12(8):1113–1119.

[57] Gjerde K, Lehmann S, Berge ME, Johansson AK, Johansson A. Oral appliance treatment in moderate and severe obstructive sleep apnoea patients non-adherent to CPAP. J Oral Rehabil 2016 Apr;43(4):249–258.

[58] De Corso E, Bastanza G, Della Marca G, Grippaudo C, Rizzotto G, Marchese MR, et al. Drug-induced sleep endoscopy as a selection tool for mandibular advancement therapy by oral device in patients with mild to moderate obstructive sleep apnoea. Acta Otorhinolaryngol Ital 2015 Dec;35(6):426–432.

[59] Okuno K, Sasao Y, Nohara K, Sakai T, Pliska BT, Lowe AA, et al. Endoscopy evaluation to predict oral appliance outcomes in obstructive sleep apnoea. Eur Respir J 2016 May;47(5):1410–1419.

[60] Johnson KG, Johnson DC. Treatment of sleep-disordered breathing with positive airway pressure devices: technology update. Med Devices (Auckl) 2015 Oct 23;8:425–437.

[61] Gao W, Jin Y, Wang Y, Sun M, Chen B, Zhou N, et al. Is automatic CPAP titration as effective as manual CPAP titration in OSAHS patients? A meta-analysis. Sleep Breath 2012 Jun;16(2):329–340.

http://dx.doi.org/10.5772/66816

[62] Ip S, D'Ambrosio C, Patel K, Obadan N, Kitsios GD, Chung M, et al. Auto-titrating versus fixed continuous positive airway pressure for the treatment of obstructive sleep apnea: a systematic review with meta-analyses. Syst Rev 2012 Mar 8;1:20–4053–1–20.

[63] Xu T, Li T, Wei D, Feng Y, Xian L, Wu H, et al. Effect of automatic versus fixed continuous positive airway pressure for the treatment of obstructive sleep apnea: an up-to-date meta-analysis. Sleep Breath 2012 Dec;16(4):1017–1026.

[64] Blau A, Minx M, Peter JG, Glos M, Penzel T, Baumann G, et al. Auto bi-level pressure relief-PAP is as effective as CPAP in OSA patients—a pilot study. Sleep Breath 2012 Sep;16(3):773–779

[65] Carlucci A, Ceriana P, Mancini M, Cirio S, Pierucci P, D'Artavilla Lupo N, et al. Efficacy of bilevel-auto treatment in patients with obstructive sleep apnea not responsive to or intolerant of continuous positive airway pressure ventilation. J Clin Sleep Med 2015 Sep 15;11(9):981–985.

[66] Gentina T, Fortin F, Douay B, Dernis JM, Herengt F, Bout JC, et al. Auto bi-level with pressure relief during exhalation as a rescue therapy for optimally treated obstructive sleep apnoea patients with poor compliance to continuous positive airways pressure therapy—a pilot study. Sleep Breath 2011 Jan;15(1):21–27.

[67] Powell ED, Gay PC, Ojile JM, Litinski M, Malhotra A. A pilot study assessing adherence to auto-bilevel following a poor initial encounter with CPAP. J Clin Sleep Med 2012 Feb 15;8(1):43–47.

[68] Wozniak DR, Lasserson TJ, Smith I. Educational, supportive and behavioural interventions to improve usage of continuous positive airway pressure machines in adults with obstructive sleep apnoea. Cochrane Database Syst Rev. 2014 Jan 8;(1):CD007736.

[69] Deleanu OC, Pocora D, Mihalcuta S, Ulmeanu R, Zaharie AM, Mihaltan FD. Influence of smoking on sleep and obstructive sleep apnea syndrome. Pneumologia 2016 Jan-Mar;65(1):28–35.

[70] Krishnan V, Dixon-Williams S, Thornton JD. Where there is smoke...there is sleep apnea: exploring the relationship between smoking and sleep apnea. Chest 2014 Dec;146(6):1673–1680.

[71] Bosi M, De Vito A, Gobbi R, et al. The importance of obstructive

[72] sleep apnoea and hypopnea pathophysiology for customized therapy. Eur Arch Otorhinolaryngol. 2016 Jul 28.

[73] Vroegop AV, Vanderveken OM, Boudewyns AN, Scholman J, Saldien V, Wouters K, et al. Drug-induced sleep endoscopy in sleep-disordered breathing: report on 1,249 cases. Laryngoscope 2014 Mar;124(3):797–802.

[74] Edwards BA, Wellman A, Sands SA, Owens RL, Eckert DJ, White DP, et al. Obstructive sleep apnea in older adults is a distinctly different physiological phenotype. Sleep 2014 Jul 1;37(7):1227–1236.

[75] Chowdhuri S, Quan SF, Almeida F, Ayappa I, Batool-Anwar S, Budhiraja R, et al. An official American Thoracic Society Research statement: impact of mild obstructive sleep apnea in adults. Am J Respir Crit Care Med 2016 May 1;193(9):e37–54.

[76] Chung F, Memtsoudis SG, Ramachandran SK, Nagappa M, Opperer M, Cozowicz C, et al. Society of anesthesia and sleep medicine guidelines on preoperative screening and assessment of adult patients with obstructive sleep apnea. Anesth Analg 2016 Aug;123(2):452–473.

[77] Colvin LJ, Collop NA. Commercial motor vehicle driver obstructive sleep apnea screening and treatment in the United States: an update and recommendation overview. J Clin Sleep Med 2016 Jan;12(1):113–125.

Chapter 2

Nerve and Muscle Changes in the Upper Airways of Subjects with Obstructive Sleep Apnea: Structural Basis for the Neurogenic Theory

Teresa Cobo, Emilio Macías, Covandonda Álvarez,
Alberto Álvarez-Suárez, Felix de Carlos,
Jose A. Vega and Juan Cobo

Additional information is available at the end of the chapter

http://dx.doi.org/10.5772/65438

Abstract

Obstructive sleep apnea syndrome (OSAS) is a widely diffused disease associated with specific genetics, age, gender, craniofacial and upper airways anatomy, obesity, and endocrine conditions, but not with ethnicity profiles. The so-called neurogenic neurogenic theory of OSAS postulates that the collapse of the upper airways that characterize this disease is due to peripheral nerve degeneration that leads to muscle atrophy and collapse. This review attempts to summarize the structural and functional changes in both the sensory and motor innervation of the walls of the upper air ways in patients suffering from OSAS.

Keywords: peripheral neuropathy, nerve fibers, mechanoreceptors, skeletal muscles, obstructive sleep apnea syndrome

1. Introduction

Obstructive sleep apnea syndrome (OSAS) is a common chronic disease characterized by sleep fragmentation due to apnea-hypoapnea and repeated arousal [1]. OSAS afflicts 2–4% of the population and has a strong genetic component [2]. Moreover, age, gender, craniofacial structure and the anatomy of the upper airways (UA), endocrine conditions, and obesity, but not ethnicity, are associated with OSAS [3].

The collapse of UA during sleep is the major characteristic of OSAS [4]. Two primary theories have been proposed to explain the pathophysiology of OSAS: the obstructive theory, in which muscle hypertrophy leads to airway narrowing, and the neurogenic theory, which postulates that peripheral nerve degeneration due to vibratory stretch trauma, or systemic diseases, lead to muscle atrophy and collapse [5–7]. A progressive local neurogenic lesion caused by repeated microtrauma of snoring might be a potential contribution factor for UA collapsibility [8].

The UA size and resistance are tightly regulated by neural mechanisms that control muscles and reflexes. The sensory nerve endings in the mucosa and mechanoreceptors of UA walls respond to changes in different sensory modalities (light touch, temperature, pressure, pain, muscle stretch and proprioception, water and chemical stimuli). Sensory inputs from these structures continually streams toward the central nervous system, including respiratory centers, which control UA muscles via efferent motor neural outputs [9], thus adjusting the contraction of the UA muscles during sucking, swallowing, respiration, speech, and mastication, as well as gagging, vomiting, coughing, and snoring reflexes (**Figure 1**). The structural

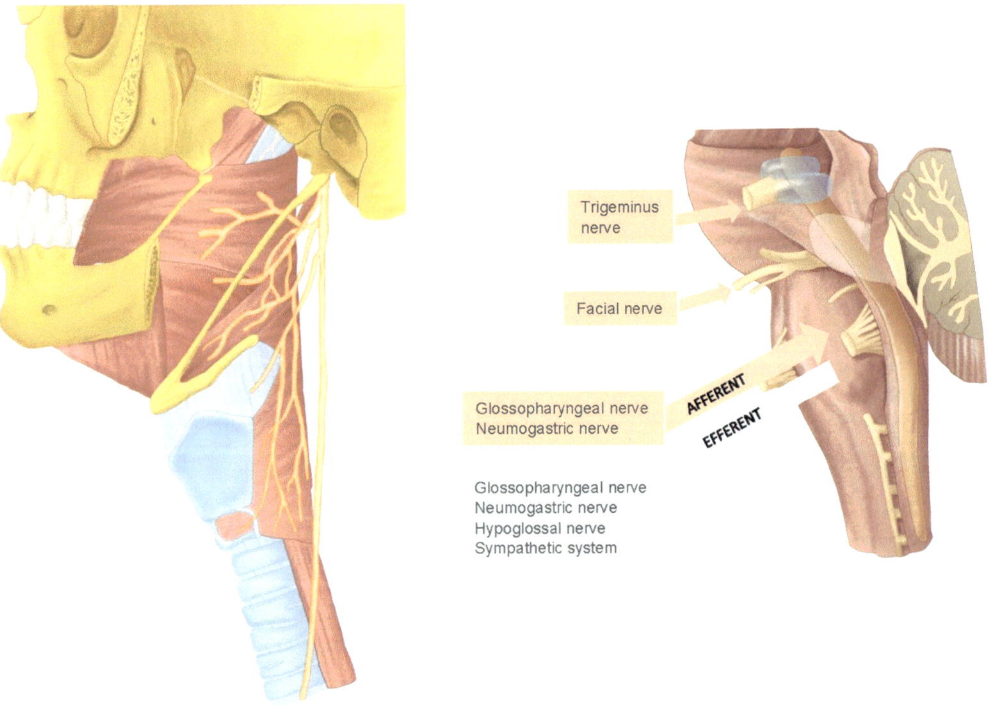

Figure 1. Schematic representation of the afferent and efferent innervation of the upper air ways. The mucosa of the nasopharynx, oropharynx, and laryngopharynx are primarily supplied by the trigeminus (maxillary division, V2), glossopharyngeal (IX), and vagus (X) cranial nerves, respectively, with a minimal contribution of the facial nerve (VII). The sensory neurons of these nerves are placed in the parent sensory ganglia and their central processes synapse within the trigeminal and tractus solitarius nuclei of the brain stem. These nuclei send the inputs to nuclei whose motoneurons are located in the pons trigeminal, facial, ambiguous, and hypoglossal nuclei, and in the anterior horn of the cervical spinal cord (C1-2). Axons from these motor neurons travel through cranial nerves V, VII, IX to XII, and the ansa cervicalis and form motor endplates that use acetylcholine for neurotransmission via nicotinic receptors to innervate innervating UA muscles (for a more detailed description of these muscles and nerves, see Massey [68]).

http://dx.doi.org/10.5772/65438

support of these reflexes consists of sensory receptors connected with sensory nerve fibers, the central synaptic connections that almost always use interneurons, and the efferent pathway composed of the motoneurons, innervating the effector organ. The effector organ in a somatic reflex is the striated muscle innervated by the α-motoneurons [10].

2. The neurological theory of OSAS and the upper airways remodeling

In the last decade of twentieth century, Woodson et al. [11] hypothesized that the pathophysiologic events that lead to the development of airway instability may be secondary to modifications in neurologic control, airway morphology, or both. Changes in sensation, muscle structure, and physiological properties of UA have been reported in patients with OSAS; these changes are referred to as airway remodeling. But whereas the structural and functional properties of muscles of OSAS patients have been extensively analyzed [5, 12–14], the motor nerve fibers and motor endplates as well as the potential role of sensory nerve impairment in OSAS have not been sufficiently investigated [15, 16]. Furthermore, the available data are heterogeneous and sometimes contradictory, because of the heterogeneity of the UA muscles, the different nerves innervating these muscles and the UA mucosae, and the differences in the methods used.

The nerve and muscle characteristics of OSAS patients may result from complex interactions of vibratory stretch trauma, inflammation, and hypoxia [8, 15–20]. It has been proposed that the repeated mechanical trauma and/or hypoxemia associated with OSA may lead to sensory and motor impairment of upper airway structures [8, 21], or that local nerve lesions due to long-standing snoring vibrations could be the basis of OSAS or its progression [17, 22, 23]. But is the neuropathy of OSAS, the cause or a consequence of the disease? It is unknown to what extent chronic intermittent hypoxemia in OSAS causes damage to the motor and sensory peripheral nerve, but muscle action potential and sensory nerve action potential amplitudes are significantly reduced in the nerves outside UA in patients with OSAS suggesting that axonal damage exists in patients with OSAS to a greater extent than previously thought [24]. On the other hand, association between OSAS and sensory neuropathy, and nerve damage outside the UA [18, 25–27], type 2 or type 1A diabetic neuropathy, and axonal subtypes of Charcot-Marie-Tooth disease [28–31] has been also demonstrated. Of particular interest is the epidemiological association between OSAS and anterior ischemic optic neuropathy [32] although a concluding rapport cannot be established [33].

Thus, there is a large body of evidence that UA neuromuscular abnormalities are frequent in OSAS patients, and these altogether support the neurogenic theory of OSAS [5–7, 34]. In recent years, multiple studies have demonstrated altered UA sensory input and abnormal UA motor function in patients with OSAS using a variety of neurophysiological and histological approaches [5, 7, 35–37], and impaired neural function is at least partly reversible with treatment for sleep apnea [27].

3. Nerve changes in OSAS

Consistent with the above data, studies on the innervation of the palate-pharyngeal region in OSAS patients have revealed both increased and decreased number of nerves in the mucosa

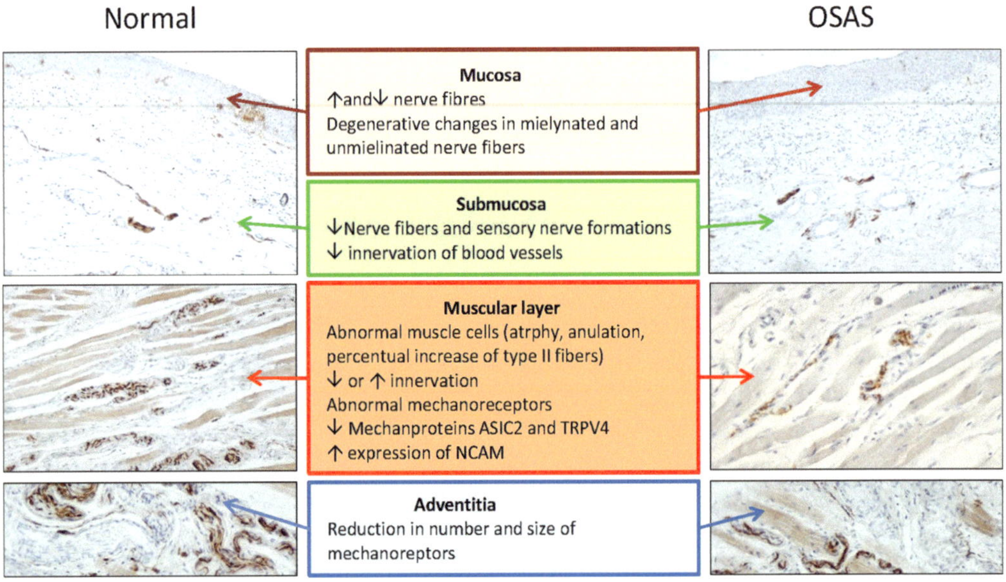

Figure 2. Main changes in nerves and muscles in OSAS patients in comparison with non-OSAS subjects. Data are based on the text and the figures are a courtesy of J.A. Vega.

and muscles [8, 13, 38, 39], as well as degenerative changes in myelinated and unmyelinated nerve fibers [40], and the degree of sensory neuropathy in UA correlates with the degree of OSAS (**Figure 2**) [41].

3.1. The afferent system: functional and structural data

If the anatomically deeper motor axons are affected by UA vibration, sensory afferents closer to the airway surface should also be impaired thus impairing normal inputs for reflex mechanisms which contribute to the upper airway function. Nevertheless, the evidence supporting sensory nerve impairment in OSA is less convincing than that for motor nerves.

The mucosal sensory function is impaired at multiple UA sites in OSAS [16]. Focal degeneration of myelinated and nonmyelinated nerve fibers, affecting Schwann cells and axons in the soft palate and uvula have been demonstrated in OSAS patients [11, 40]. In these UA zones, increase in the density of epithelial afferent nerve endings (based on the expression of substance P and calcitonin gene-related peptide) was also observed which is indicative of nerve lesion [38]. On the other hand, the afferent information from UA muscles is important in regulating the masticatory force and oromotor behaviors, but also in the response of important reflexes related to speech, swallowing, cough, vomit, or normal breathing [10, 42]. Patients with OSAS show a significant reduction in the density of nerve fibers in the submucosa as well as morphological abnormalities in mechanosensory corpuscles. Importantly, the muscle innervation of nerve fibers expressing ASIC2 and TRPV4 (regarded as two putative mechanoproteins) is also reduced in these subjects [43].

http://dx.doi.org/10.5772/65438

In addition, and consistently with the above-mentioned pathological findings, UA sensory function has been shown to be impaired in OSAS during wakefulness [13, 15, 16, 44], specially patients with OSAS have altered vibration and cold detection thresholds [45, 46]. The respiratory-related evoked potentials (RREPs) during wakefulness in OSA revealed a reduction in the amplitude but not the latency of the early RREP components [44, 47] reflecting sensory processing is reduced in the OSA patients [48]. Other studies revealed no changes [49–51].

3.2. The efferent system: functional and structural data

Data regarding the changes in motor nerves during OSAS are scarce. Motor neuron lesions and/or direct damage in the muscles [17, 41] as well a decrease [39, 43] or increase [13] in the number of nerve fibers have been reported. But most studies have focused directly on muscles.

4. Muscle changes in OSAS

Structural changes in skeletal muscles have been studied primarily in the uvula muscles and the palatopharyngeal muscle, and the reported changes are very heterogeneous. They include focal muscle atrophy and muscle bundle disruption [11, 52], prevalence of angulated muscle fibers, increased and/or reduction of muscle fibers diameter and variation in fiber type grouping [14, 23, 53–57], atrophic and hypertrophic muscle fibers [8, 52, 58], changes in mitochondria content [14], enzymatic changes [56], and increased neural cell adhesion molecule expression by muscle cells [13].

Another characteristic of the UA muscles is the high percentage disproportion of glycolytic fast twitch of type II muscle fibers compared with non-OSA control subjects [12, 14, 55, 59–62], a difference that may represent an adaptive response to mechanical strain and/or neuronal activity. In this way, the over expression of N-CAM is suggestive of collateral nerve sprouting, reflected in the hyperinnervation that present these muscles [13]. Vascular enlargement, fibrosis, edema, inflammatory cells, and infiltration have also been reported. There is also increased fat in and around the muscles of the UA in patients with OSA [63].

However, all these changes in muscle fibers are not a major contributing factor to OSAS pathogenesis in most patients [20].

In addition to the structural changes, the UA muscles also show electrophysiological changes in OSAS. Patients with OSA have higher levels of multiunit electromyographic activity (EMG) recorded in the UA muscles compared to healthy control subjects presumably secondary to neurogenic remodeling. This is characterized by chronic partial denervation of muscle fibers, with reinnervation of the orphaned muscle fibers by collateral sprouting of surviving motor axons [13, 60, 64–66]. The apparent increase in drive was ascribed to a neural compensation for a narrow UA.

Recent investigations using single motor unit techniques have shown that the motor unit potentials of upper airway muscles in OSA patients are larger in area, longer in duration, and more complex [7, 23, 37]. These changes could contribute to the increased multiunit EMG in OSAS. However, the presence of denervation and subsequent axonal sprouting may lead to changes in fine motor control such as speech [67].

5. Concluding remarks and future perspectives

The involvement of the peripheral nervous system and muscles in the pathogenesis of OSAS is now accepted. Nevertheless, large have been reported presumably due to the methodological differences used to evaluate both the pathological and functional changes in UA of patients suffering from OSAS. So, whereas some researchers found decrease in the density of nerve fibers [39, 40, 43] some others have found increased numbers of nerve fibers in the mucosa and muscles [13, 38]. These discrepancies can be related to the zones of the UA sampled or the muscles analyzed. And more importantly, no specific markers for sensory or motor nerve fibers were used in these studies. Another important aspect is the studies about the state of motor end-plates in OSAS. Thus, further studies are required to elucidate the role of upper airway sensory and motor impairment in modulating disease progression or severity.

Author details

Teresa Cobo[1,2], Emilio Macías[1,2], Covandonda Álvarez[1,2], Alberto Álvarez-Suárez[3], Felix de Carlos[2], Jose A. Vega[4*] and Juan Cobo[1,2]

*Address all correspondence to: javega@uniovi.es

1 Orthodontics Area - Instituto Asturiano de Odontología, Oviedo, Spain

2 Department of Surgery and Medical-Surgical Specialties (Section of Odontology), University of Oviedo, Spain

3 Mechanical Engineering Area – Instituto Asturiano de Odontología, Oviedo, Spain

4 Department of Morphology and Cell Biology, SINPOS Group, University of Oviedo, Spain

References

[1] Dempsey JA, Veasey SC, Morgan BJ, O'Donnell CP. Pathophysiology of sleep apnea. Physiol Rev. 2010; 90:47–112. DOI: 10.1152/physrev.00043.2008.

[2] Paiva T, Attarian H. Obstructive sleep apnea and other sleep-related syndromes. Handb Clin Neurol. 2014; 119:251–271. DOI: 10.1016/B978-0-7020-4086-3.00018-7.

[3] Ralls FM, Grigg-Damberger M. Roles of gender, age, race/ethnicity, and residential socioeconomics in obstructive sleep apnea syndromes. Curr Opin Pulm Med. 2012; 18: 568–573. DOI: 10.1097/MCP.0b013e328358be05.

[4] Eckert DJ, Malhotra A. Pathophysiology of adult obstructive sleep apnea. Proc Am Thorac Soc. 2008; 5: 144–153. DOI: 10.1513/pats.200707-114MG.

[5] Saboisky JP, Butler JE, Gandevia SC, Eckert DJ. Functional role of neural injury in obstructive sleep apnea. Front Neurol. 2012; 3: 95. DOI: 10.3389/fneur.2012.00095. eCollection 2012.

[6] Tsai YJ, Ramar K, Liang YJ, Chiu PH, Powell N, Chi CY, Lung TC, Wen-Yang Lin W, Tseng PJ, Wu MY, Chien KC, Weaver EM, Lee FP, Lin CM, Chen KC, Chiang RP. Peripheral neuropathology of the upper airway in obstructive sleep apnea syndrome. Sleep Med Rev. 2013; 17:161–168. DOI: 10.1016/j.smrv.2012.05.005.

[7] Saboisky JP, Butler JE, Luu BL, Gandevia SC. Neurogenic changes in the upper airway of obstructive sleep apnoea. Curr Neurol Neurosci Rep. 2015; 15:12. DOI: 10.1007/s11910-015-0537-1.

[8] Friberg D, Ansved T, Borg K, Carlsson-Nordlander B, Larsson H, Svanborg E. Histological indications of a progressive snorer disease in an upper airway muscle. Am J Respir Crit Care Med. 1998; 157:586–593. DOI: 10.1164/ajrccm.157.2.96–06049.

[9] Horner RL. Neural control of the upper airway: integrative physiological mechanisms and relevance for sleep disordered breathing. Compr Physiol. 2012; 2: 479–535. DOI: 10.1002/cphy.c110023.

[10] Miller AJ. Oral and pharyngeal reflexes in the mammalian nervous system: their diverse range in complexity and the pivotal role of the tongue. Crit Rev Oral Biol Med. 2002; 13: 409–425. DOI: 10.1177/154411130201300505.

[11] Woodson BT, Garancis JC, Toohill RJ. Histopathologic changes in snoring and obstructive sleep apnea syndrome. Laryngoscope. 1991; 101:1318–1322. DOI: 10.1002/lary.5541011211.

[12] Lindman R, Stal PS. Abnormal palatopharyngeal muscle morphology in sleep-disordered breathing. J Neuro Sci. 2002; 195: 11–23. DOI: 10.1016/S0022-510X(01)00676-1.

[13] Boyd JH, Petrof BJ, Hamid Q, Fraser R, Kimoff RJ. Upper airway muscle inflammation and denervation changes in obstructive sleep apnea. Am J Respir Crit Care Med. 2004; 170: 541–546. DOI: 10.1164/rccm.200308-1100OC.

[14] Stål PS, Lindman R, Johansson B. Capillary supply of the soft palate muscles is reduced in long-term habitual snorers. Respiration. 2009; 77:303–310. DOI: 10.1159/000197975.

[15] Kimoff RJ, Sforza E, Champagne V, Ofiara L, Gendron D. Upper airway sensation in snoring and obstructive sleep apnea. Am J Respir Cri. Care Med. 2001; 164: 250–255. DOI: 10.1164/ajrccm.164.2.2010012.

[16] Nguyen AT, Jobin V, Payne R, Beauregard J, Naor N, Kimoff RJ. Laryngeal and velopharyngeal sensory impairment in obstructive sleep apnea. Sleep. 2005; 28: 585–593.

[17] Friberg D. Heavy snorer's disease: a progressive local neuropathy. Acta Otolaryngol. 1999; 119: 925–933.

[18] Mayer P, Dematteis M, Pépin JL, Wuyam B, Veale D, Vila A, Lévy P. Peripheral neuropathy in sleep apnea: a tissue marker of the severity of nocturnal desaturation. Am J Respir Crit Care Med. 1999; DOI: 159:213–219. 10.1164/ajrccm.159.1.9709051.

[19] Donald F1, Esdaile JM, Kimoff JR, Fitzcharles MA. Musculoskeletal complaints and fibromyalgia in patients attending a respiratory sleep disorders clinic. J Rheumatol. 1996; 23:1612–1616.

[20] Eckert DJ, Saboisky JP, Jordan AS, Malhotra A. Upper airway myopathy is not important in the pathophysiology of obstructive sleep apnea. J Clin Sleep Med. 2007; 3: 570–573.

[21] Petrof BJ, Hendricks JC, Pack AI. Does upper airway muscle injury trigger a vicious cycle in obstructive sleep apnea? A hypothesis. Sleep. 1996; 19:465–471.

[22] Svanborg E. Upper airway nerve lesions in obstructive sleep apnea. Am J Respir Crit Care Med. 2001; 164: 187–189. DOI: 10.1164/ajrccm.164.2.2105010c.

[23] Svanborg E. Impact of obstructive apnea syndrome on upper airway respiratory muscles. Respir Physiol Neurobiol. 2005; 147: 263–272. DOI:10.1016/j.resp.2005.06.012.

[24] Mihalj M, Lušić L, Đogaš Z. Reduced evoked motor and sensory potential amplitudes in obstructive sleep apnoea patients. J Sleep Res. 2016; 25: 287–295. DOI: 10.1111/jsr.12368.

[25] Dematteis M, Pepin JL, Jeanmart M, Deschaux C, Labarre-Vila A, Levy P. Charcot-Marie-Tooth disease and sleep apnoea syndrome: a family study. Lancet 2001; 357: 267–272. DOI:10.1016/S0140-6736(00)03614-X.

[26] Lüdemann P, Dziewas R, Soros P, Happe S, Frese A. Axonal polyneuropathy in obstructive sleep apnoea. J Neurol Neurosurg Psychiatr. 2001; 70: 685–687. DOI:10.1136/jnnp.70.5.685.

[27] Dziewas R, Schilling M, Engel P, Boentert M, Hor H, Okegwo A, Ludemann P, Ringelstein EB, Young P. Treatment for obstructive sleep apnoea: effect on peripheral nerve function. J Neurol Neurosurg Psychiatr. 2007; 78: 295–297. DOI: 10.1136/jnnp.2006.102806.

[28] Tahrani AA, Ali A, Raymond NT, Begum S, Dubb K, Mughal S, Jose B, Piya MK, Barnett AH, Stevens MJ. Obstructive sleep apnea and diabetic neuropathy: a novel association in patients with type 2 diabetes. Am J Respir Crit Care Med. 2012; 186: 434–441. DOI: 10.1164/rccm.201112-2135OC.

[29] Aurora RN, Punjabi NM. Obstructive sleep apnoea and type 2 diabetes mellitus: a bidirectional association. Lancet Respir Med. 2013; 1: 329–338. DOI: 10.1016/S2213-2600(13)70039-0.

[30] Boentert M, Knop K, Schuhmacher C, Gess B, Okegwo A, Young P. Sleep disorders in Charcot-Marie-Tooth disease type 1. J Neurol Neurosurg Psychiatry. 2013; 85: 319–325. DOI: 10.1136/jnnp-2013-305296.

[31] Fujihara K, Kodama S, Horikawa C, Yoshizawa S, Sugawara A, Hirasawa R, Shimano H, Yachi Y, Suzuki A, Hanyu O, Sone H. The relationship between diabetic neuropathy and sleep apnea syndrome: a meta-analysis. Sleep Disord. 2013: 150371. DOI: 10.1155/2013/150371.

[32] Aptel F, Khayi H, Pépin JL, Tamisier R, Levy P, Romanet JP, Chiquet C. Association of nonarteritic ischemic optic neuropathy with obstructive sleep apnea syndrome: consequences for obstructive sleep apnea screening and treatment. JAMA Ophthalmol. 2015; 133: 797–804. DOI: 10.1001/jamaophthalmol.2015.0893.

[33] Wu Y, Zhou LM, Lou H, Cheng JW, Wei RL. The association between obstructive sleep apnea and nonarteritic anterior ischemic optic neuropathy: a systematic review and meta-analysis. Curr Eye Res. 2015; 7: 1–6. DOI: 10.3109/02713683.2015.1075221.

[34] Levý P, Pépin JL, Dematteis M. Pharyngeal neuropathy in obstructive sleep apnea: where are we going? Am J Respir Crit Care Med. 2012; 185: 241–243. DOI: 10.1164/rccm.201111-1992ED.

[35] Guilleminault C, Huang YS, Kirisoglu C, Chan A. Is obstructive sleep apnea syndrome a neurological disorder? A continuous positive airway pressure follow-up study. Ann Neurol. 2005; 58: 880–887. DOI: 10.1002/ana.20654.

[36] Guilleminault C, Ramar K. Neurologic aspects of sleep apnoea: is obstructive sleep apnoea a neurologic disorder? Semin Neurol. 2009; 29: 68–71. DOI: 10.1055/s-0029-1237122.

[37] Saboisky JP, Stashuk DW, Hamilton-Wright A, Carusona AL, Campana LM, Trinder J, Eckert DJ, Jordan AS, McSharry DG, White DP, Nandedkar S, David WS, Malhotra A. Neurogenic changes in the upper airway of patients with obstructive sleep apnea. Am J Respir Crit Care Med. 2012; 185: 322–329. DOI: 10.1164/rccm.201106-1058OC.

[38] Friberg D, Gazelius B, Hökfelt T, Nordlander B. Abnormal afferent nerve endings in the soft palatal mucosa of sleep apnoics and habitual snorers. Regul Pept. 1997; 71: 29–36. DOI:10.1016/S0167-0115(97)01016-1.

[39] De Bellis M, Pagni F, Ronchi S, Limonta G, Gorla S, Nicoletti G, Cucci M, Di Bella C, Vicini C. Immunohistochemical and histomorphometric study of human uvula innervation: a comparative analysis of non-snorers versus apneic snorers. Sleep Breath. 2012; 16: 1033–1040. DOI: 10.1007/s11325-011-0597-7.

[40] Bassiouny A, Nasr S, Mashaly M, Ayad E, Qotb M, Atef A. Electron microscopy study of peripheral nerves in the uvulae of snorers and obstructive sleep apnoea patients. J Laryngol Otol. 2009; 123: 203–207. DOI: 10.1017/S0022215108002971.

[41] Sunnergren O, Broström A, Svanborg E. Soft palate sensory neuropathy in the pathogenesis of obstructive sleep apnea. Laryngoscope 2011; 121: 451–456. DOI: 10.1002/lary.21371.

[42] De Carlos F, Cobo J, Macías E, Feito J, Cobo T, Calavia MG, García-Suárez O, Vega JA. The sensory innervation of the human pharynx: searching for mechanoreceptors. Anat Rec (Hoboken). 2013; 296: 1735–1746. DOI: 10.1002/ar.22792.

[43] De Carlos F, Cobo J, Macías E, Feito J, González M, Cobo T, Fernández-Mondragón MP, García-Suárez O, Vega JA. Reduced innervation in the human pharynx in patients with obstructive sleep apnea. Histol Histopathol. 2015; 30: 865–874. DOI: 10.14670/HH-11-593.

[44] Akay M, Leiter JC, Daubenspeck JA. Reduced respiratory-related evoked activity in subjects with obstructive sleep apnea syndrome. J Appl Physiol. 2003; 94: 429–438. DOI: 10.1152/japplphysiol.00018.2001.

[45] Larsson H, Carlsson-Nordlander B, Lindblad LE, Norbeck O, Svanborg E. Temperature thresholds in the oropharynx of patients with obstructive sleep apnea syndrome. Am Rev Respir Dis. 1992; 146: 1246–1249. DOI: 10.1164/ajrccm/146.5_Pt_1.1246.

[46] Hagander L, Harlid R, Svanborg E. Quantitative sensory testing in the oropharynx: a means of showing nervous lesions in patients with obstructive sleep apnea and snoring. Chest. 2009; 136: 481–489. DOI: 10.1378/chest.08-2747.

[47] Grippo A, Carrai R, Romagnoli I, Pinto F, Fanfulla F, Sanna A. Blunted respiratory-related evoked potential in awake obstructive sleep apnoea subjects: a NEP technique study. Clin. Neurophysiol. 2011; 122: 1562–1568. DOI: 10.1016/j.clinph.2011.01.005.

[48] Afifi L, Guilleminault C, Colrain IM. Sleep and respiratory stimulus specific dampening of cortical responsiveness in OSAS. Respir Physiol Neurobiol. 2003; 136: 221–234. DOI: 10.1016/S1569-9048(03)00084-3.

[49] Donzel-Raynaud C, Redolfi S, Arnulf I, Similowski T, Straus C. Abnormal respiratory-related evoked potentials in untreated awake patients with severe obstructive sleep apnoea syndrome. Clin Physiol Funct Imaging. 2009; 29: 10–17. DOI: 10.1111/j.1475-097X.2008.00830.x.

[50] Eckert DJ, Lo YL, Saboisky JP, Jordan AS, White DP, Malhotra A. Sensori-motor function of the upper airway muscles and respiratory sensory processing in untreated obstructive sleep apnea. J Appl Physiol. 2011; 111: 1644–1653. DOI: 10.1152/japplphysiol.00653.2011.

[51] Vakulin A, Catcheside PG, Baulk SD, Antic NA, van den Heuvel CJ, Banks S, McEvoy RD. Auditory evoked potentials remain abnormal after CPAP treatment in patients with severe obstructive sleep apnoea. Clin Neurophysiol. 2012; 123: 310–317. DOI: 10.1016/j.clinph.2011.07.004.

[52] Edstrom L, Larsson H, Larsson L. Neurogenic effects on the palatopharyngeal muscle in patients with obstructive sleep apnoea: a muscle biopsy study. J Neurol Neurosurg Psychiatr. 1992; 55: 916–920.

[53] Smirne S, Iannaccone S, Ferini-Strambi L, Comola M, Colombo E, Nemni R. Muscle fibre type and habitual snoring. Lancet. 1991; 337: 597–599.

[54] Ferini-Strambi LJ, Smirne S, Moz U, Sferrazza B, Iannaccone S. Muscle fibre type and obstructive sleep apnea. Sleep Res Online 1998; 1: 24–27.

[55] Series F, Simoneau JA, St Pierre S. Muscle fiber area distribution of musculus uvulae in obstructive sleep apnea and non-apneic snorers. Int J Obes Relat Metab Disord. 2000; 24: 410–415.

[56] Sauleda J, Garcia-Palmer FJ, Tarraga S, Maimo A, Palou A, Agusti AG. Skeletal muscle changes in patients with obstructive sleep apnoea syndrome. Respir Med. 2003; 97: 804–810. DOI: 10.1016/S0954-6111(03)00034-9.

[57] Molina FD, Santos FC, Falleiros LR Jr, Goloni-Bertollo EM, Felisbino SL, Justulin LA Jr, Maniglia JV, Taboga SR. Microscopical evaluation of extracellular matrix and its relation to the palatopharyngeal muscle in obstructive sleep apnea. Microsc Res Tech. 2011; 74: 430–439. DOI: 10.1002/jemt.20927

[58] Stål PS, Johansson B. Abnormal mitochondria organisation and oxidative activity in palate muscles of long-term snorers with obstructive sleep apnea. Respiration. 2012; 83: 407–417. DOI: 10.1159/000336040.

[59] Series F, Cote C, Simoneau JA, Gelinas Y, St Pierre S, Leclerc J, Ferland R, Marc I. Physiologic, metabolic, and muscle fiber type characteristics of musculus uvulae in sleep apnea hypopnea syndrome and in snorers. J Clin Invest. 1995;95: 20–25. DOI: 10.1172/JCI117640.

[60] Series F, Wang W, Similowski T. Corticomotor control of the genioglossus in awake OSAS patients: a transcranial magnetic stimulation study. Respir Res. 2009; 10: 74. DOI: 10.1186/1465-9921-10-74.

[61] Saboisky JP, Butler JE, McKenzie DK, Gorman RB, Trinder JA, White DP, Gandevia SC. Neural drive to human genioglossus in obstructive sleep apnoea. J Physiol. 2007; 585: 135–146. DOI: 10.1113/jphysiol.2007.139584.

[62] Vuono IM, Zanoteli E, de Oliveira AS, Fujita RR, Pignatari SS, Pizarro GU, de Cássia Pradelle-Hallinan ML, Moreira GA. Histological analysis of palatopharyngeal muscle from children with snoring and obstructive sleep apnea syndrome. Int J Pediatr Otorhinolaryngol. 2007; 71: 283–290. DOI: 10.1016/j.ijporl.2006.10.019.

[63] Berger G, Gilbey P, Hammel I, Ophir D. Histopathology of the uvula and the soft palate in patients with mild, moderate, and severe obstructive sleep apnea. Laryngoscope. 2002; 112: 357–363. DOI: 10.1097/00005537-200202000-00028.

[64] Mezzanotte WS, Tangel DJ, White DP. Influence of sleep onset on upper-airway muscle activity in apnea patients versus normal controls. Am J Respir Crit Care Med. 1996; 153: 1880–1887. DOI: 10.1164/ajrccm.153.6.8665050.

[65] Fogel RB, Malhotra A, Giora P, Edwards JK, Beauregard J, Shea SA, White DP. Genioglossal activation in paitents with obstructive sleep apnea versus control subjects. Am J Respir Crit Care Med. 2001; 164: 2025–2030. DOI: 10.1164/ajrccm.164.11.2102048.

[66] Gonzalez-Forero D, Portillo F, Sunico CR, Moreno-Lopez B. Nerve injury reduces responses of hypoglossal motoneurones to baseline and chemoreceptor-modulated inspiratory drive in the adult rat. J Physiol. 2004; 57: 991–1011. DOI: 10.1113/jphysiol.2003.059972.

[67] Goldshtein E, Tarasiuk A, Zigel Y. Automatic detection of obstructive sleep apnea using speech signals. IEEE Eng Med Biol Mag. 2011; 58: 1373–1382. DOI: 10.1109/TBME.2010.2100096.

[68] Massey BT. Physiology of oral cavity, pharynx, and upper esophageal sphincter. GI Motility Online. 2006; DOI: 10.1038/gimo2.

Chapter 3

Usefulness of Artificial Neural Networks in the Diagnosis and Treatment of Sleep Apnea-Hypopnea Syndrome

Daniel Álvarez, Ana Cerezo-Hernández,
Graciela López-Muñiz, Tania Álvaro-De Castro,
Tomás Ruiz-Albi, Roberto Hornero and
Félix del Campo

Additional information is available at the end of the chapter

http://dx.doi.org/10.5772/66570

Abstract

Sleep apnea-hypopnea syndrome (SAHS) is a chronic and highly prevalent disease considered a major health problem in industrialized countries. The gold standard diagnostic methodology is in-laboratory nocturnal polysomnography (PSG), which is complex, costly, and time consuming. In order to overcome these limitations, novel and simplified diagnostic alternatives are demanded. Sleep scientists carried out an exhaustive research during the last decades focused on the design of automated expert systems derived from artificial intelligence able to help sleep specialists in their daily practice. Among automated pattern recognition techniques, artificial neural networks (ANNs) have demonstrated to be efficient and accurate algorithms in order to implement computer-aided diagnosis systems aimed at assisting physicians in the management of SAHS. In this regard, several applications of ANNs have been developed, such as classification of patients suspected of suffering from SAHS, apnea-hypopnea index (AHI) prediction, detection and quantification of respiratory events, apneic events classification, automated sleep staging and arousal detection, alertness monitoring systems, and airflow pressure optimization in positive airway pressure (PAP) devices to fit patients' needs. In the present research, current applications of ANNs in the framework of SAHS management are thoroughly reviewed.

Keywords: sleep apnea-hypopnea syndrome, pattern recognition, automated biomedical signal processing, artificial neural networks, multilayer perceptron, feed-forward back-propagation, Bayes theory

1. Introduction

In their daily practice, physicians must frequently decide a definitive diagnosis or the most suitable treatment using several variables from multiple clinical data sources, which is a highly complex task. A huge amount of valuable healthcare-related information is currently available, from symptoms reported by the patient and details stored in their clinical history to biochemical data and outcomes from biomedical recordings or medical images. In this context, machine learning methods are essential to maximize the usefulness of medical data in order to expedite decisions and avoid misdiagnosis. In the last decades, the increasing development of computers and artificial intelligence has led to the use of decision support expert systems in the common clinical practice of several fields of medicine [1, 2]. The huge number of studies published in the context of biomedical engineering during the last years clearly shows this trend.

Bayesian theory was one of the first mathematical frameworks used to implement decision support systems. Regarding the classification of an item, according to the Bayes' decision rule, the predicted class must be the one that maximizes *a posteriori* probability in order to minimize the classification error. A major goal is to model the statistical characteristics of the problem under study, leading to expert systems able to assist physicians in decision-making processes. Among pattern recognition algorithms, conventional statistical classifiers, such as discriminant analysis [3] or logistic regression (LR) [4], and more recently artificial neural networks (ANNs) [5], have been widely applied. The widely known statistical classifiers assume that the class density function of input data is known *a priori*. Assumptions such as normal distribution, homoscedasticity, linearity, independency, or stationarity decrease the complexity of the classifier, minimize the classification error, and improve the performance. Nevertheless, these assumptions are not always consistent in real-world pattern classification problems, especially when working with limited datasets. Conversely, when using ANNs, no assumptions are made about the probability density functions of input features and the training data is used directly to optimize the decision rule [6]. Nevertheless, ANNs are characterized by a complex design stage. Both statistical and ANNs approaches have its advantages and limitations. However, the ability to model complex nonlinear problems, which are very common in biological systems, have made ANNs widely used in medical applications.

The first attempt to model information processing in biological systems by means of ANNs was carried out by McCulloch and Pitts in 1943 [7]. Since then, ANN-based algorithms have significantly evolved and their use in the field of medicine has increased considerably, particularly since the late 1990s. Some computer programs in the context of statistical medicine already include ANNs among their functionalities, which has contributed to increase their use in medical research. Nevertheless, "neural network" remains frequently a confusing term for many healthcare-related researchers. The implementation of an ANN has to be carried out by means of advanced software and some expertise is required to set up properly the user-dependent input parameters. However, once designed, they are reliable and easy to use tools, even by nontrained personnel. In addition, once optimized, the computational time is small, which is a major feature in order to speed up decision making.

http://dx.doi.org/10.5772/66570

Sleep research and particularly sleep-related breathing disorders (SBD) is a field in which the application of automated pattern recognition algorithms has increased exponentially during the last years due to the need for automating their complex diagnostic processes. Particularly challenging is the management of sleep apnea-hypopnea syndrome (SAHS). The gold standard technique for SAHS diagnosis is in-lab nocturnal polysomnography (PSG). During PSG, several neuromuscular and cardiorespiratory signals (up to 32 biomedical recordings) are monitored and stored for subsequent interpretation by trained personnel, which is a highly complex and time-consuming task [8]. In addition, accessibility to diagnosis and treatment is limited due to insufficient resources, both human (trained specialists) and technical (specialized sleep units), which have led to large waiting lists [9]. In this context, automated computer-aided diagnosis systems have emerged as very useful tools to deal with complex rules involving several biomedical recordings simultaneously, in order to expedite diagnosis and treatment [10–12]. Among all the machine learning-based tools, ANNs have been widely applied in the context of SAHS and merit a thorough analysis.

In order to analyze the usefulness of ANNs in the management of SAHS, an exhaustive review of the studies published during the past decade has been carried out. The review is structured as follows. First, the most relevant tasks regarding the ANNs learning process are outlined in Section 2. In this regard, some user-dependent decisions involving the ANN design and major issues concerning the training and testing processes are detailed. Second, in Section 3, the most relevant applications of ANNs are analyzed, including automated diagnosis, sleep staging, and treatment monitoring.

2. Artificial neural networks

ANNs are mathematical models inspired in the information processing capabilities of the nervous system designed to accomplish a predetermined task specified by the user [13, 14]. They were built to implement useful brain functions into a pattern recognition algorithm, such as parallel processing, distributed memory/storage, and environmental flexibility. ANNs are characterized by a fast and effective processing, learned from a preceding training process. During the learning or training stage, a wide set of known representative samples are used in order to model the statistical properties of the problem under study and accordingly compose the structure of the network. **Figure 1** illustrates a common network architecture of interconnected nodes arranged in layers simulating the brain's neuronal synapses.

The following advantages can be obtained when ANNs are applied for pattern recognition problems: (i) no prior assumptions about the data distribution are made as ANNs adjust themselves to the particular problem constrains during the learning process [15], (ii) ANNs are universal estimators able to match any function with arbitrary accuracy [16], and (iii) they are nonlinear algorithms able to model real-world complex relationships [15].

There are two major classes of ANNs: feedforward multilayered networks and radial basis function (RBF) networks. Both types of ANNs are capable of approximating any continuous functional mapping by means of several units (neurons) arranged in different layers [17]. The

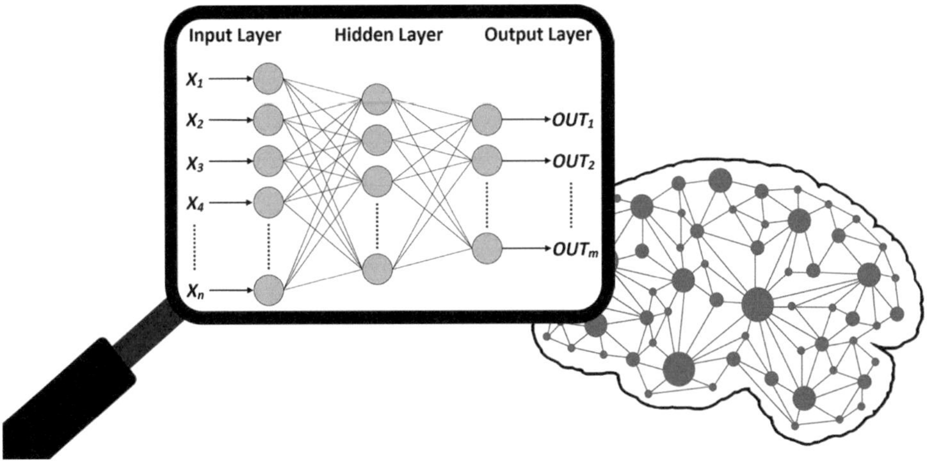

Figure 1. Common network architecture of interconnected nodes arranged in three layers (input, hidden, and output) simulating the brain's neuronal synapses.

main difference is the way hidden units are activated, i.e., how the input data is used to compute the output of each unit. In feedforward ANNs, there is a fixed (usually nonlinear) activation function, whereas in RBF ANNs, the activation of each unit depends on the radial distance (typically Euclidean) between the input vector and a prototype vector (center) [18].

The multilayer perceptron (MLP) is the most widely used feedforward ANN in computer-aided medical research. Indeed, feedforward networks, particularly MLP, are the most popular ANN in the framework of SAHS management [19–21]. A particular implementation of MLP networks involving Bayesian inference during the learning process (BY-MLP), which increase the generalization ability and allow for relevance analysis of input variables, has demonstrated to be useful in this context [22]. Similarly, probabilistic neural networks (PNN), which also integrates the Bayes' theory into the learning process, have been recently applied in the SAHS diagnosis problem [23]. In addition, RBF ANNs [24, 25], such as learning vector quantization (LVQ), which is a precursor of self-organizing maps using the Hebbian learning-based approach [26, 27]; fuzzy neural networks (FNN), which incorporate the fuzzy inference system (FIS) into the learning process [26, 28, 29]; self-organizing maps (SOM) and adaptive resonance theory (ART) models, which are likely the most common unsupervised ANNs [30, 31]; and recurrent neural networks (RNN), which allow for closed-loop connections between units (feedback) [32], have been also applied in the framework of automated SAHS management.

Next, an overview of the conventional multilayered network architecture is provided, as well as the most important issues regarding the design, training, and validation stages common to all approaches in the ANN-based framework. **Figure 2** shows a flow diagram summarizing these stages.

2.1. Network design: architecture of a neural network

The so-called neuron is the basic element within an ANN, which comprises its elementary mathematical functions [17]. ANNs are composed of multiple interconnected nodes arranged in different levels or layers leading to a massive parallel structure. The first level is called the

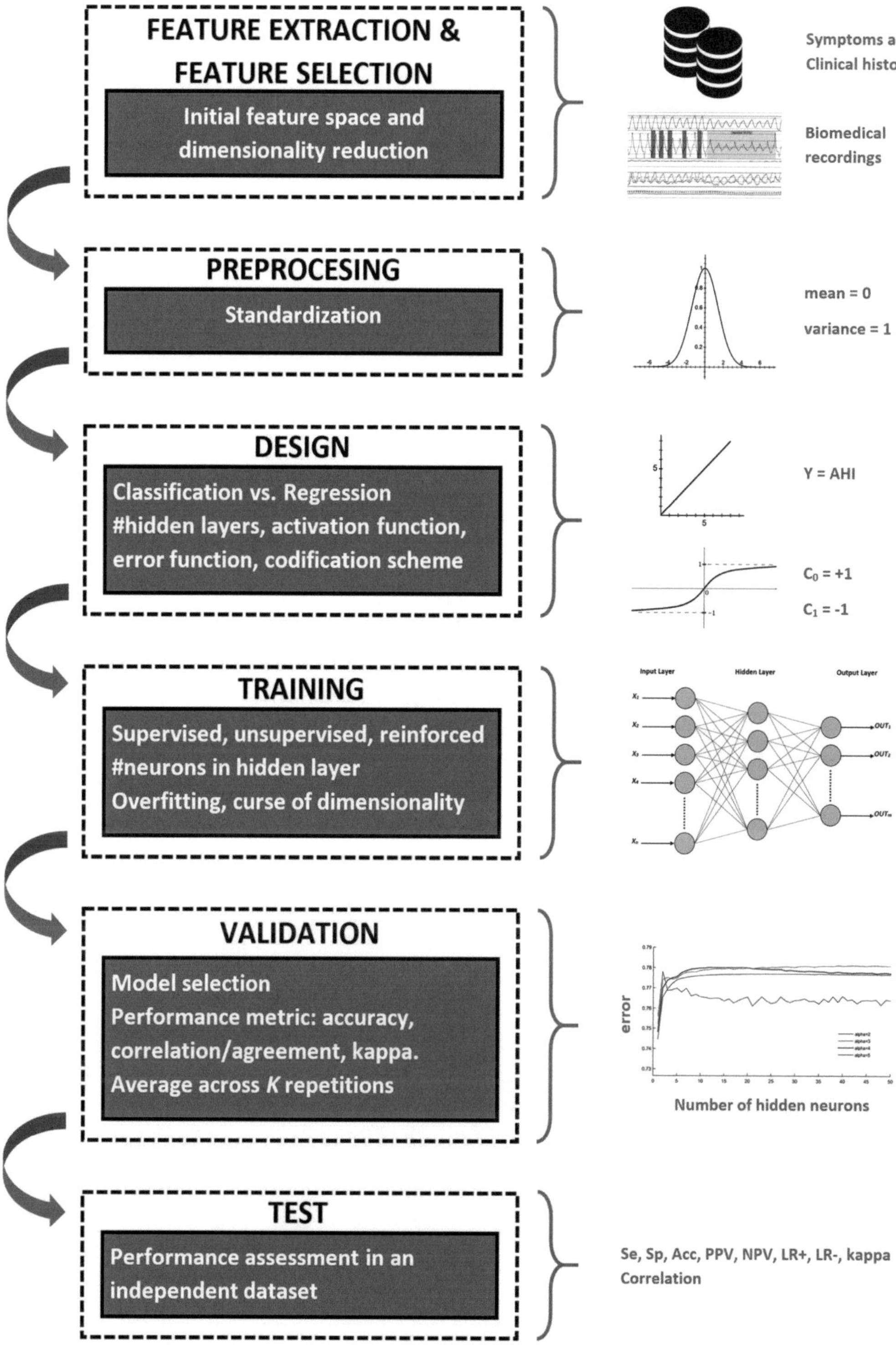

Figure 2. Flow diagram summarizing the training, validation, and test stages, as well as the most important issues involved in the design of an ANN.

input layer. Neurons in the input layer process directly the feature vectors or patterns that feed the ANN. Similarly, each output from every neuron in a layer feeds neurons composing the subsequent layer, leading to a distributed complex structure. The last level of the network, whose nodes provide the output of the ANN, is called the output layer. The remaining internal levels are called hidden layers. Both the number of hidden layers and the number of nodes are flexible and are determined during the learning process. The feedforward architecture is the most widely used, where each neuron in a layer is connected to every neuron on the next layer but neither connections between units in the same level nor closed-loops (feedback) are allowed. Therefore, data is always moving forward from one layer to the next, i.e., from the input to the output.

There is not a predetermined network architecture known to be *a priori* the best for any problem under study in terms of performance. The mathematical operation accomplished by each neuron is always the same. Therefore, the functionality of the ANN, i.e., the way in which a particular problem is addressed, is determined by the strength of the link between each pair of neurons. This strength is characterized by the coefficients of the ANN, the so-called weights, which are optimized during the training stage. Similar to the process of memory, weights represent the information stored in the network, whereas the optimization procedure represents the learning process or statistical inference [18].

As aforementioned, the structure of an ANN depends on the number of hidden layers, the number of neurons per layer, and the connectivity strength among them. Regarding the number of levels, it is common to construct ANNs with a single hidden layer because it has been demonstrated that this architecture is able to achieve universal approximation [33]. This is a user-dependent decision, whereas the number of neurons and the connectivity degree (weights) are both determined automatically during the learning process. Regarding the number of nodes in the hidden layer, it is commonly optimized by means of a hold-out or cross-validation approach using the data in a training dataset. In this regard, it is supposed that the complex the problem, the higher the number of neurons. Notwithstanding, even a small network with a reduced number of nodes can model complex problems and reach high prediction ability. In addition, the following design issues must be addressed before the learning process [17]: the output coding scheme, the error function used in the network training, and the activation function of neurons in the hidden and output layers. The hyperbolic tangent function is a common activation function for neurons in the hidden layer since it has been demonstrated that it provides fast convergence of training algorithms [13, 17]. **Figure 3** shows a common schema of a single neuron (perceptron) with a sigmoid activation function. Regarding the learning process, the scale conjugate gradient (SCG) is a common method for updating the adjustable parameters of the ANN (weights and biases) during the training stage.

2.1.1. Classification and regression approaches

According to the mathematical nature of the output, ANNs can be applied to address two main kinds of problems: classification and regression. Regarding the classification approach, the goal of the ANN is to estimate the class membership for an input feature pattern among a

http://dx.doi.org/10.5772/66570

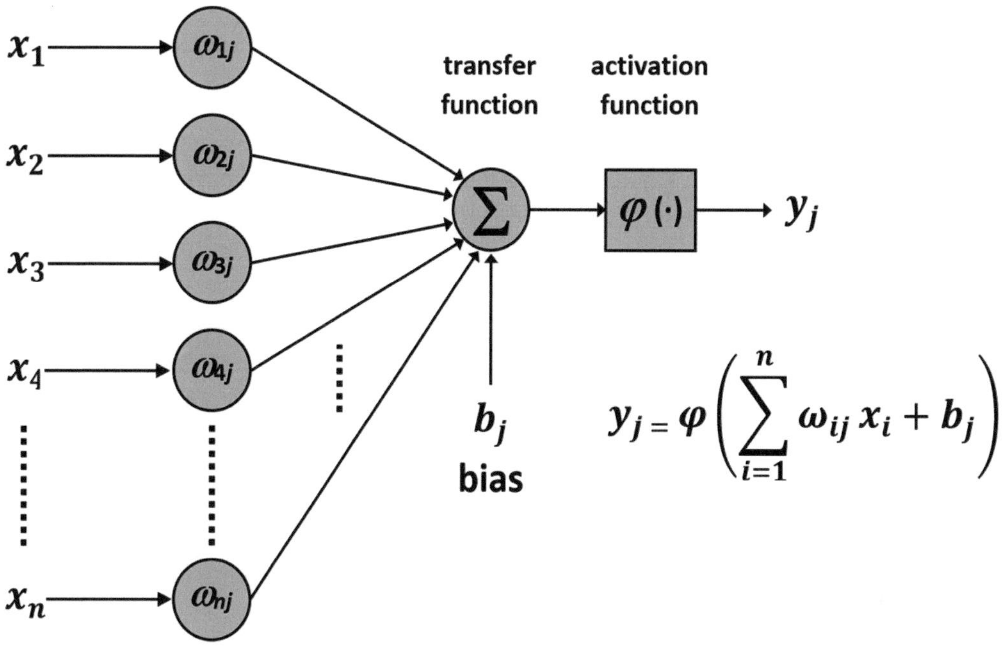

Figure 3. Scheme of a perceptron. A nonlinear activation function φ(·) is applied to the weighted sum of the input features (x_n) and the bias term (b_j) in order to compute the output (y_k).

set of predefined discrete categories. Conversely, in a regression task, the goal of the ANN is to estimate a continuous variable.

In the context of binary classification problems, an output layer with just a single neuron is needed. Regarding, for instance, a 2-class SAHS diagnosis problem, all input patterns are assigned to one of two mutually exclusive classes: SAHS positive (class C_0 or positive class) or SAHS negative (class C_1 or negative class). A possible target coding scheme would be the following: $t = 0$ for the positive class and $t = 1$ for the negative class. This architecture can be used also in regression problems, where the variable to be approximated is unidimensional and continuous. In the context of SAHS diagnosis, the goal of a regression ANN could be to estimate the apnea-hypopnea index (AHI).

Due to a highly flexible architecture, most of the ANNs can be used to model both classification and regression problems by just modifying certain design characteristics [17]. The main difference between classification and regression ANNs is linked with the nature of the function to be approximated. The output of an ANN is provided in terms of probability in a classification task while it is an estimate of a continuous variable in a regression context. Accordingly, optimization procedures differ from one approach to another. Regarding a binary classification approach, the activation function of the output neuron could be a nonlinear function with output values ranging [0, 1], e.g., sigmoid functions such as the logistic or the hyperbolic tangent. In this regard, the network output can be interpreted as the probability that the input feature pattern belongs to one class or another according to the Bayes' theorem. Conversely, addressing a regression task, the network output values must be continuous and nonnegative. Therefore, a linear activation function ranging [0, ∞) would be suitable.

Regarding the error function governing the learning process, the cross-entropy error function is widely used in the context of binary classification, whereas the sum-of-squares error function is commonly used for regression purposes [17].

2.1.2. Standardization of input patterns

Normalization of input feature values is an important task in nonlinear pattern recognition methods [34]. Bounded similar input magnitudes are needed to accomplish suitable weight initialization. Input patterns are composed of features parameterizing different properties of the problem under study, e.g., the influence of recurrent apnea events typical of SAHS on cardiorespiratory signals. Usually, several features of different nature are involved in order to obtain as much information as possible, e.g., sociodemographic, anthropometric, clinical, and/or variables from automated feature extraction algorithms. Therefore, their values may differ significantly and thus they must be normalized. In this regard, simple linear rescaling can be used to standardize (zero mean and unit variance) the magnitudes of each input feature by subtracting its mean and dividing by its standard deviation.

2.2. The training process: learning the problem under study

Training is the most important stage when working with ANNs. The aim of the training process is to adapt the ANN to the problem under study by computing some adjustable parameters. The training or learning process can be (i) supervised, in which the learning process is guided by a static mapping between input patterns and known targets; (ii) reinforced, in which a performance function assesses the accuracy of the current output instead of knowing the actual target values; and (iii) unsupervised, in which ANNs adapt themselves to input patterns with no kind of feedback [35]. In the context of medical decision support systems, the supervised approach is the most widely used. When using supervised learning, it is essential to know the target or actual output value for a wide set of input patterns. The dataset of examples used during the learning stage is referred to as the training set. According to this training input-output pairs, the network weights are tuned to fit the input to its corresponding target. It is important that the training set would be large enough to represent fairly the problem under study.

The backpropagation learning is the most commonly used methodology for updating weights in feedforward ANNs due to its computational efficiency [17]. Using this approach, all weights are updated every time an input pattern is fed from the training dataset in order to minimize an error function. First, the network weights are initialized randomly. During a supervised learning process, the training samples (input-target pairs) are fed into the network and the error function is computed, i.e., the difference between the estimated output value and the desired target according to a predefined suitable function. Then, the values of the network weights are modified in order to minimize the error. This procedure is repeated throughout several iterations, which are set by the user. Once the training process is finished, all network weights already have a fix value, i.e., there is a single optimized ANN able to carry out the task for which it was designed.

2.2.1. *Generalization ability and the problem of overfitting*

Once optimized, an ANN is able to process new input patterns independent of the training dataset. In this regard, it is noteworthy that the goal of the training stage must be to build a general statistical model of the problem under study rather than to learn data samples from a particular training set. This is an essential characteristic common to all pattern recognition techniques and it is required to achieve good generalization ability. Generalization accounts for the ability to make good predictions for new unknown inputs [17].

In addition to the user's capability to accomplish appropriate design and optimization procedures, the performance or generalization ability of an ANN is influenced by three main factors [13, 36]: (i) the size and completeness of the training dataset, i.e., whether the learning samples account for all the variability of the environment or problem of interest; (ii) the number of adjustable parameters in the model; and (iii) the complexity of the problem under study. The nature of the problem or model complexity is linked with the number of adjustable parameters in the ANN (network weights) and it cannot be controlled. Theoretically, the harder the problem, the more complex the ANN. In this regard, it is important to achieve a compromise between the generalization ability and complexity. An ANN with a small number of parameters, i.e., low flexibility, may lead to an underfitted model, insufficient to reach high generalization. On the contrary, an ANN with a large number of weights may lead to an overfitted model that matches a particular training dataset, resulting in poor generalization. Underfitting can be avoided by increasing the flexibility, whereas overfitting requires the training set to grow accordingly to the network complexity [13].

In the same way, the optimization of an ANN is closely related to the bias-variance trade-off. A too simple or inflexible model will have a large bias and may lead to underfitting. Conversely, models with a high variance provide high flexibility but could adapt to the noise present in the training set, leading to overfitting. Bias and variance are both complementary characteristics and thus the best generalization is obtained when a compromise between the conflicting requirements of small bias and small variance is achieved [15, 17].

A way to reduce both bias and variance simultaneously is to increase the number of training samples. As a result, model complexity increases, which minimizes the bias. At the same time, constrains imposed by the training data will be more rigorous, thereby also reducing variance. As mentioned earlier, to achieve this goal the size of the training set should increase in accordance with model complexity [17]. Nevertheless, this requirement cannot always be achieved in real-world applications because the size of the training set is usually fixed and limited. Therefore, finding the optimum model complexity is a major issue. In order to deal with this optimization problem, a new trade-off arises: simpler models are preferred but smoothing mapping is needed to prevent from poor generalization [13, 17]. In this regard, regularization techniques allow the ANN to control the effective complexity of the model by reducing the number of adjustable parameters during the training set. Weight decay and early stopping are common approaches of regularization. Weight decay is probably the most widely used, consisting on adding a penalty term to the error function in order to penalize complex mappings.

An additional issue regarding the training sample size is called the course of dimensionality [17]. This term refers to the relationship between the size of the training set and the dimension of the feature space, i.e., the number of variables in the input feature vector. The course of dimensionality states that the number of training samples needed to characterize the underlying problem grows exponentially as the number of input features increases. Therefore, the size of the training dataset must also increase according to the input space dimension in order to enhance generalization ability and avoid overfitting [18].

As previously stated, the size of the training set in real-world applications is fixed and usually limited, especially in the field of medicine. In this regard, dimensionality reduction techniques contribute to address the problem of overfitting due to the curse of dimensionality. An ANN fed with fewer input features needs to optimize fewer parameters (weights) and these are more likely to be properly characterized by a limited training dataset. The aim of dimensionality reduction algorithms is to compose a reduced subset of the most significant features governing a model. To achieve this goal, a fitness metric (relevancy, redundancy, completeness, or accuracy, among others) is used to obtain the optimum feature subset. There are several feature selection methodologies but principal component analysis and stepwise feature selection are likely the most widely used in medical applications.

2.3. Validation and test processes: model selection and performance assessment

In order to estimate the actual prediction ability of an ANN, the learning, model selection, and performance assessment stages must be carried out using independent datasets, i.e., the so-called training, validation, and test datasets. The goal of model selection is to obtain the optimum network configuration by comparing the performance of several ANNs with different values of the design parameters, i.e., number of neurons in the hidden layer and usually the regularization parameter. The hold-out method is commonly used for this purpose because it avoids a biased estimation of the results [36]. In the hold-out method, the initial population/dataset is split into three independent groups for training, validation, and testing purposes. The network weights are adjusted in the training set for different configurations of the adjustable parameters specified by the researcher, i.e., multiple ANNs are really trained, whereas the performance of each individual ANN is computed in the validation set to determine the optimum ANN for the problem under study. Since there is a random initialization of weights, the training process is frequently repeated several times to avoid a potential bias linked with this arbitrary decision. Thus, the performance metric for model selection from the validation set is averaged across all the repetitions. Nevertheless, this procedure can lead also to some overfitting so the selected optimum ANN has to be further assessed in an independent test set composed of unseen data samples [17].

It is worth to notice that, unfortunately, several studies from the literature do not implement a suitable validation of their proposed methodology, providing biased overoptimistic results [37]. On the other hand, sometimes the initial dataset is not large enough to properly derive the three independent subpopulations. In such cases, cross-validation techniques allow for training and validating the models in the same training set without biasing the selection of the optimum model. Bootstrap, leave-one-out, and *k*-fold cross-validation are common algorithms to deal with small populations under study.

3. Clinical applications of NNs in the context of sleep apnea-hypopnea syndrome

ANNs have been applied to model problems in several fields, such as industrial processes optimization, economic and financial modeling, chemistry, physics, biology, or medicine, among others [38–42]. In the framework of SAHS management, automated expert systems based on ANNs have been mainly applied to classify patients suspected of suffering from SAHS (binary classification: no SAHS vs. SAHS), to categorize the severity of the disease (multiclass classification: no SAHS, mild, moderate, and severe), to estimate the AHI (regression of a continuous variable), to detect and quantify respiratory events (normal breathing vs. apneic), and to categorize apneic events (central, obstructive, and mixed). ANNs have been also used to implement automated sleep staging and arousal detection, which are very useful functionalities incorporated in current commercial software applications for sleep analysis. In addition, ANNs play an important role in alertness monitoring systems and they are already integrated in positive airway pressure (PAP)-based treatment devices to fit user's airflow needs, which are major issues for patients suffering from SBDs.

Most research in the field of SAHS focus on binary classification in order to determine the presence or absence of the disease. Similarly, some studies also applied ANNs for multiclass classification in order to characterize SAHS severity according to predefined discrete categories. Conversely, despite of its higher information about the severity of the disease, only a few studies have been carried out to estimate the AHI using a regression approach (continuous function).

Regarding the nature of the input data, ANNs aimed at assisting in SAHS diagnosis first used anthropometric and clinical features to compose input patterns [19, 43]. However, the increasing research in the context of biomedical signal processing allows physicians to derive essential information directly from signals monitored during the PSG [44]. In this regard, blood oxygen saturation (SpO_2) from oximetry and heart rate variability (HRV) from electrocardiogram (ECG) are the most widely used. In addition, airflow from both thermistor and nasal pressure, abdominal and chest movements, snoring sounds, and EEG have been also studied. Alternatively, in order to avoid sleep studies, automated signal processing of speech recordings and even image analysis for facial recognition have been also assessed as an alternative to PSG-derived signals to assist in the detection of SAHS.

The main goal of computer-aided tools for SAHS management is to simplify and speed up the diagnostic methodology, in order to alleviate large waiting lists and increase accessibility of patients to diagnostic resources. Current research focuses on analyzing a reduced set of biomedical recordings, which are preferably obtained at patient's home using existing commercial portable devices. Therefore, powerful tools are needed to obtain as much information as possible from this reduced subset of signals. In this regard, ANNs allow researchers to manage several features derived from the signals under study and thus they are suitable and reliable tools to help physicians in the diagnosis of SAHS. In order to obtain complementary information, different automated signal processing methods have been applied, such as common statistics (mean, median, variance, skewness, kurtosis), time domain analyses (detection and quantification of respiratory events), frequency domain analyses (Fourier analysis, time-frequency maps, wavelet transform, bispectrum), and/or nonlinear methods (entropy measures, Poincaré plots, complexity measures), among others, both individually or jointly.

3.1. SAHS diagnosis by means of ANNs

ANNs were first used in the context of SAHS detection in the late 1990s, when Kirby et al. [43] and El-Solh et al. [19] carried out retrospective analyses aimed at designing ANNs based on clinical and anthropometric variables from patients showing clinical suspicion of SAHS. **Table 1** summarizes the main characteristics of significant studies carried out during the last decade focused on applications of ANNs aimed at assisting in SAHS diagnosis. In the study by Kirby et al. [43], 23 clinical variables fed a generalized regression neural network (GRNN), which is a kind of RBF network, for binary classification (SAHS vs. no SAHS). The authors reported 98.9% sensitivity, 80.0% specificity, and 91.3% accuracy (86.8–95.8, CI 95%). Similarly, El-Solh et al. [19] used clinical and anthropometric variables in order to estimate the AHI by means of a MLP ANN. Using cutoffs of 10, 15, and 20 events per hour (e/h) for a positive diagnosis of SAHS, the sensitivity-specificity pairs were 94.9–64.7%, 95.3–60.0%, and 95.5–73.4%, respectively. Both studies achieved significantly high sensitivity but poor to moderate specificity, which is a common trend of pattern recognition techniques in the context of SAHS.

Recent studies have built updated predictive models based on anthropometric and clinical data, since characteristics of patients referred nowadays to sleep units have changed compared to those of patients in the last decade. In this regard, Su et al. [45] proposed the multiclass Mahalanobis-Taguchi system (MMTS) and used both anthropometric information and questionnaire data in order to classify patients into normal subjects or mild, moderate, or severe SAHS patients. Additionally, LR, conventional feed-forward backpropagation FFBB and LVQ ANNs, support vector machines (SVM), C4.5 decision tree (DT), and rough set (RS) were also applied for comparison purposes. The proposed MMTS significantly outperformed the competing classifiers, reaching an average accuracy of 84.38% (normal: 87.50%; mild: 66.67%; moderate: 100%; severe: 83.33%). Particularly, FFBB and LVQ ANNs reached 34.04% (normal: 25.00%; mild: 33.33%; moderate: 11.11%; severe: 66.70%) and 47.22% (normal: 50.00%; mild: 16.67%; moderate: 22.22%; severe: 100%) overall accuracy, respectively. Similarly, in a recent study carried out by Wang et al. [27] several automated classifiers fed with anthropometric and questionnaire-based variables were also assessed to predict SAHS. The authors propose a novel classifier based on fuzzy decision trees (FDT) to detect SAHS. In addition, LR, ANNs (backpropagation and LVQ), a SVM, and a conventional DT were used as benchmarks for comparison purposes. The proposed FDT achieved the highest performance (81.82% accuracy, 0.554 *kappa*, and 0.673 geometric mean). However, a synthetic oversampling approach (SMOTE) was used to deal with the common imbalance between SAHS positive and SAHS negative classes, which was not used in the remaining benchmark methods. Without SMOTE, FDTs slightly outperformed the backpropagation ANN (48.22% vs. 47.53% accuracy, 0.186 vs. 0.175 *kappa*, and 0.300 vs. 0.288 geometric mean), whereas the highest precision was achieved by the conventional LR approach (49.57% accuracy, 0.207 *kappa*, and 0.320 geometric mean). Karamanli et al. recently assessed a MLP ANN trained to classify healthy and SAHS patients using sex, age, BMI, and snoring status as input variables, reporting 86.6% accuracy [21]. Nevertheless, it is important to highlight that input features derived automatically from

Author (year) [Ref.]	ANN model	Purpose	Target function/ class(es)	Input variables	Performance metrics
Kirby et al. (1999) [43]	GRNN	Classification (binary)	No SAHS vs. SAHS (AHI ≥10 e/h)	Clinical	98.9% Se 80.0% Sp 91.3% Acc
El-Solh et al. (1999) [19]	MLP	Regression	AHI estimation	Clinical and anthropometric	CC = 0.852 cutoff 10 e/h 94.9% Se - 64.7% Sp cutoff 15 e/h 95.3% Se - 60.0% Sp cutoff 20 e/h 95.5% Se - 73.4% Sp
Su et al. (2012) [45]	MMTS LR FFBB LVQ SVM DT RS	Classification (4-class)	Normal/mild/ moderate/severe	Anthropometric and questionnaire data	84.38% average Acc 55.33% average Acc 34.04% average Acc 47.22% average Acc 53.82% average Acc 63.54% average Acc 13.20% average Acc
Wang et al. (2016) [27]	FFBB LVQ	Classification (4-class)	No SAHS/mild/ moderate/severe	Anthropometric and questionnaire data	47.5% Acc, 0.145 *k*, 0.288 g-mean 43.4% Acc, 0.181 *k*, 0.280 g-mean
Karamanli et al. (2016) [21]	MLP	Classification (binary)	No SAHS vs. SAHS (AHI ≥10 e/h)	Sex, age, BMI, snoring status	86.6% Acc
Polat et al. (2008) [29]	FFBB ANFIS	Classification (binary)	No SAHS vs. SAHS (AHI ≥ 5 e/h)	In-lab PSG-derived	100% Se, 93.5% Sp, 95.1% Acc, 0.96 AUC
Ghandeharioun et al. (2015) [30]	SOM	Classification (4-class)	No SAHS/mild/ moderate/severe	In-lab PSG-derived and anthropometric	94.2% Se, 97.8% Sp, 96.5% Acc
Marcos et al. (2008) [20]	MLP	Classification (binary)	No SAHS vs. SAHS (AHI ≥10 e/h)	Nonlinear features from SpO_2	89.8% Se, 79.4% Sp, 85.5% Acc
Marcos et al. (2008) [24]	RBF-KM RBF-FCM RBF-OLS	Classification (binary)	No SAHS vs. SAHS (AHI ≥10 e/h)	Nonlinear features from SpO_2	89.4% Se, 81.4% Sp, 86.1% Ac 86.6% Se, 81.9% Sp, 84.7% Acc 89.8% Se, 79.4% Sp, 85.5% Acc
Almazaydeh et al. (2012) [46]	MLP	Classification (binary)	Healthy vs. SAHS (AHI ≥5 e/h) Physionet	ODI3, delta index, CTM from SpO_2	87.5% Se, 100% Sp, 93.3% Acc
Marcos et al. (2010) [22]	MLP BY-MLP	Classification (binary)	No SAHS vs. SAHS (AHI ≥10 e/h)	Statistical, spectral, and nonlinear features from SpO_2	86.4% Se, 62.8% Sp, 76.8% Acc 87.8% Se, 82.4% Sp, 85.6% Acc
Morillo et al. (2012) [47]	BY-MLP	Classification (binary)	No SAHS *vs.* SAHS (AHI ≥10 e/h)	Time, stochastic, spectral, and nonlinear features from SpO_2	92.4% Se, 95.9% Sp, 93.9% Acc

Author (year) [Ref.]	ANN model	Purpose	Target function/ class(es)	Input variables	Performance metrics
Huang et al. (2015) [26]	FFBB LVQ ANFIS	Classification (binary)	No SAHS vs. SAHS (AHI ≥5 e/h)	ODI4 from SpO_2	88.0% Se, 93.3% Sp, 90.7% Acc 80.7% Se, 79.3% Sp, 80.0% Acc 90.7% Se, 86.0% Sp, 88.3% Acc
Khandoker et al. (2009) [23]	SVM LDA KNN PNN	Classification (binary)	Healthy vs. SAHS (AHI ≥5 e/h) Physionet	Wavelet decomposition of HRV and EDR from ECG	100% Se, 100% Sp, 100% Acc 90% Se, 100% Sp, 93% Acc 80% Se, 90% Sp, 83% Acc 80% Se, 50% Sp, 70% Acc
Khandoker et al. (2008) [48]	FFBB	Classification (binary)	Apneic vs. Normal Hypopnea vs. Apnea Obstructive vs. Central	ECG	87.6% Se, 95.5% Sp, 95.1% Acc 86.1% Se, 78.7% Sp, 83.4% Acc 93.7% Se, 99.2% Sp, 98.9% Acc
Acharya et al. (2011) [49]	FFBB	Classification (3-class)	Normal/apnea/ hypopnea	Nonlinear measures from ECG	95.0% Se, 100% Sp, 99.1% Acc (normal) 88.0% Se, 90.0% Sp, 96.5% Acc (apnea) 80.0% Se, 89.5% Sp 87.8% Acc (hypopnea)
Lweesky et al. (2011) [50]	FFBB	Classification (binary)	Normal breathing vs. apnea epochs	P-wave features from ECG	90.0% Se, 94.2% Sp, 92.0% Acc
Mendez et al. (2009) [51]	FFBB	Classification (binary)	Normal breathing vs. apnea (AHI ≥5 e/h)	Time and spectral features from RRi and QRS area time series	89.0% Se, 86.0% Sp, 88.0% Acc (m-by-m) 100% Acc (record)
Nguyen et al. (2014) [52]	ANN SVM Ensemble	Classification (binary)	Normal sleep vs. sleep apnea epochs	HRV complexity by means of RQA	85.6% Se, 79.1% Sp, 83.2% Acc 93.7% Se, 65.9% Sp, 84.1% Acc 86.4% Se, 83.5% Sp, 85.3% Acc
Fiz et al. (2010) [53]	MLP	Classification (binary)	No SAHS vs. SAHS AHI ≥5 e/h AHI ≥15 e/h	Time and spectral features from snoring recordings	87.0% Se, 71.0% Sp 80.0% Se, 90.0% Sp
Nguyen and Won (2015) [54]	f-MLP MLP	Classification (binary)	Normal breathing vs. snoring	Spectral content snoring recordings	96.0% overall Acc 82.0% overall Acc
Tagluk et al. (2011) [55]	MLP	Classification (binary)	Normal vs. SAHS EEG epochs	Bispectral analysis of EEG	94.1% Se, 98.2% Sp, 96.2% Acc

Author (year) [Ref.]	ANN model	Purpose	Target function/ class(es)	Input variables	Performance metrics
Liu et al. (2008) [31]	ART2	Classification (binary)	Healthy vs. SAHS subjects (AHI ≥5 e/h)	EEG energy in theta (Fourier transform) and pupil size	91.0% Acc
Lin et al. (2006) [28]	FFBB	Classification (binary)	No SAHS vs. SAHS epochs	EEG power in delta, theta, alpha, and beta using DWT	69.64% Se, 44.44% Sp
Akşahin et al. (2012) [56]	FFBB RBF DTD	Classification (3-class)	Obstructive/central/ healthy patients	Coherence and mutual information of EEG	0.1450 MRAE error 0.3692 MRAE error 0.2282 MRAE error
Fontela et al. (2005) [57]	BY-MLP	Classification (3-class)	Obstructive/central/ mixed	Wavelet decomposition of thoracic effort	83.78% Acc (overall) 80.90% Acc (obstr.) 89.95% Acc (centr.) 80.48% Acc (mixed)
Tagluk et al. (2010) [58]	FFBB	Classification (3-class)	Obstructive/central/ mixed	Wavelet decomposition of abdominal effort	78.50% Acc (overall) 73.42% Acc (obstr.) 94.23% Acc (centr.) 66.16% Acc (mixed)
Berdiñas et al. (2012) [59]	Ensemble ANNs	Classification (3-class)	Obstructive/central/ mixed	Wavelet decomposition of thoracic effort	90.27% Acc (overall) 94.62% Acc (obstr.) 95.47% Acc (centr.) 90.45% Acc (mixed)
Weinreich et al. (2008) [60]	FFBB	Classification (4-class)	OA/OH/CSR/normal breathing	Spectral entropy of airflow	91.5% Acc (overall) 90.2% Se, 90.9% Sp (OA vs. CSR) 91.3% Se, 94.6% Sp (OH vs. normal)
Várady et al. (2002) [61]	FFBB	Classification (3-class)	Normal/apnea/ hypopnea	IRA and IRI from airflow and RIP	93.0% Acc (overall) 98.4% Se, 94.0% Sp (normal) 78.7% Se, 91.0% Sp (hypopnea) 97.0% Se, 88.7% Sp (apnea)
Belal et al. (2011) [62]	MLP	Classification (binary)	Non-apneic *vs.* apneic event	Correlation and PCA of HR, RR, and SpO_2	81.8% Se, 75.8% Sp, 76.8% Acc
Marcos et al. (2012) [63]	MLP	Regression	AHI estimation	Spectral and nonlinear features from SpO_2	ICC = 0.91 cutoff 5 e/h 91.8% Se–58.8% Sp cutoff 10 e/h 89.6% Se–81.3% Sp cutoff 15 e/h 94.9% Se–90.9% Sp

Author (year) [Ref.]	ANN model	Purpose	Target function/ class(es)	Input variables	Performance metrics
Gutiérrez-Tobal et al. (2013) [25]	MLP RBF	Regression	AHI	Statistical, spectral, nonlinear features from airflow	ICC = 0.849 ± 0.002 cutoff 10 e/h 92.5% Se, 89.5% Sp, 91.5% Acc ICC = 0.748 ± 0.037 cutoff 10 e/h 92.5% Se, 57.9% Sp, 81.4% Acc
de Silva et al. (2011) [64]	FFBB	Regression	AHI	Pitch, formant, and structure-based features from snoring sounds and the neck circumference	Cutoff 15 e/h 91 ± 6% Se, 89 ± 5% Sp Cutoff 30 e/h 86 ± 9% Se, 88 ± 5% Sp
de Silva et al. (2012) [65]	FFBB	Regression	AHI	Pitch, formant, and structure-based features from snoring sounds and the neck circumference	Female, AHI ≥ 15 e/h 91 ± 10% Se, 88 ± 5% Sp Male, AHI ≥ 15 e/h 91 ± 6% Se, 89 ± 5% Sp Comb., AHI ≥ 15 e/h 84 ± 10% Se, 83 ± 13% Sp
Emoto et al. (2012) [66]	MLP	Regression	Breathing sound signal	Preceding samples of the breathing signal	89.2% average Se 87.4% average Sp

Notes: Se: sensitivity; Sp: specificity; Acc: accuracy; e/h: events per hour; CC: correlation coefficient; *k*: kappa coefficient; g-mean: geometric-mean; ICC: intra-class correlation coefficient; GRNN: generalized regression neural network; SAHS: sleep apnea-hypopnea syndrome; AHI: apnea-hypopnea index; MLP: multilayer perceptron; MMTS: multiclass Mahalanobis-Taguchi system; LR: logistic regression; FFBB: feed-forward back-propagation; LVQ: learning vector quantization; SVM: support vector machine; DT: decision tree; RS: rough set; ANFIS: adaptive network-based fuzzy inference system; SOM: self-organizing maps; BMI; body mass index; RBF: radial basis function; KM: *k*-means; FCM; fuzzy *c*-means; OLS: orthogonal least squares; SpO_2: blood oxygen saturation from nocturnal oximetry; ODI3: oxygen desaturation index of 3%; CTM: central tendency measure (nonlinear); BY-MLP: Bayesian training MLP neural network; PNN: probabilistic neural network; ODI4: oxygen desaturation index of 4%; HRV: heart rate variability; EDR: ECG-derived respiration; RRi: R-to-R interval time series; QRS: QRS complex from the ECG; *k*-NN: *k* nearest neighbors; RQA: recurrence quantification analysis; f-MLP: correlational filter MLP; ART2: modified adaptive resonance theory ANN; DWT: discrete wavelet transform; OA: obstructive apnea; OH: obstructive hypopnea; CSR: Cheyne-Stokes respiration; DTD: distributed time-delay neural network; MRAE: mean relative absolute error; IRA: instantaneous respiration amplitude; IRI: instantaneous respiration interval; RIP: respiratory inductance plethysmography; HR: heart rate; RR: respiratory rate.

Table 1. Performance and the most relevant characteristics of the studies using ANNs in the context of SAHS classification, event detection, and AHI regression.

cardiorespiratory and/or neuromuscular signals have been used predominantly, while anthropometric and clinical variables have been used marginally.

In the study by Polat et al. [29], different expert systems were assessed to classify patients with suspicion of SAHS using clinical features derived from in-lab polysomnography, including the arousal index and the AHI. A FFBB ANN reached 100% sensitivity, 93.55%

specificity, 95.12% accuracy, and 0.96 AUC, slightly lower and more unbalanced than a DT-based classifier (91.67% sensitivity, 96.55% specificity, 95.12% accuracy, and 0.97 AUC). This work assessed the usefulness of different expert systems in the context of SAHS, although using input variables computed from the whole PSG study limits its ability as screening test for the disease. Similarly, Ghandeharioun et al. [30] trained a 4-class SOM to classify patients suspected of suffering from SAHS into healthy, mild, moderate, and severe categories using PSG-derived and anthropometric variables. The proposed algorithm reached 94.2% sensitivity, 97.8% specificity, and 96.5% accuracy, although neither validation nor test stages were described.

Regarding SAHS diagnosis by means of ANNs, the SpO_2 signal from nocturnal oximetry is probably the most widely used biomedical data source. In the study by Marcos et al. [20], approximate entropy (ApEn), central tendency measure (CTM), and Lempel-Ziv complexity were applied to the SpO_2 nocturnal profile to estimate irregularity, variability, and complexity, respectively. These nonlinear measures composed the input feature patterns to feed a MLP ANN for SAHS binary classification. A sensitivity of 89.8%, specificity of 79.4%, and accuracy of 85.5% were obtained in an independent test set, significantly improving the diagnostic performance of conventional oximetric indices. The same authors reached similar diagnostic performance using a RBF ANN in the same context [24]: average accuracies of 86.1 ± 1.1% (89.4 ± 1.6% sensitivity, 81.4 ± 1.7% specificity), 84.7±1.2% (86.6 ± 2.8% sensitivity, 81.9 ± 2.0% specificity), and 85.5 ± 0.0% (89.8 ± 0.0% sensitivity, 79.4 ± 0.0% specificity) were achieved using *k*-means, fuzzy *c*-means, and orthogonal least squares kernels, respectively. An MLP ANN was also assessed in the study by Almazaydeh et al. [46] to perform binary classification. The ANN was fed with the conventional oxygen desaturation index of 3% (ODI3), the delta index, and the CTM from overnight oximetry recordings, reaching 87.5% sensitivity, 100% specificity, and 93.3% accuracy in a test set from the publicly available *PhysioNet* dataset.

Bayesian training has been applied to deal with overfitting of ANNs. In addition, Bayesian inference also allows the user to measure quantitatively the influence of each input feature in the output of the model. The effectiveness of this approach was assessed in the study by Marcos et al. [22]. A sensitivity of 87.76%, specificity of 82.39%, and accuracy of 85.58% were reached, significantly improving the performance achieved using the conventional maximum likelihood criterion (86.42% sensitivity, 62.83% specificity, and 76.81% accuracy). Similarly, Sánchez-Morillo et al. [47] applied a feedforward probabilistic ANN to classify patients into SAHS negative or SAHS positive using time, stochastic, spectral, and nonlinear features from nocturnal SpO_2 recordings. A sensitivity of 92.42%, specificity of 95.92%, and accuracy of 93.91% were reached in a single training set using leave-one-out cross-validation. In a recent study by Huang et al. [26], the automated analysis of the oxygen desaturation index of 4% (ODI4) from oximetry by means of a DT was proposed as an abbreviated method for SAHS screening. In this work, the authors assessed several pattern recognition techniques for automated diagnosis, including some ANNs, such as conventional backpropagation, (LVQ), and adaptive network-based fuzzy inference system (ANFIS). The proposed DT reached 98.67% sensitivity, 90.67 specificity, and 94.67% accuracy, outperforming backpropagation (88.00% sensitivity, 93.33% specificity, 90.67% accuracy), ANFIS (90.67% sensitivity, 86.00% specificity,

88.33% accuracy), and LVQ (80.67% sensitivity, 79.33% specificity, 80.00% accuracy) ANNs. In this study, conventional LR and *k*-nearest neighbors (*k*-NN) combined with genetic algorithms (GAs) and particle swarm optimization (PSO) also outperformed ANNs.

ECG recordings have been also widely used to assist in SAHS diagnosis. In the study by Khandoker et al. [23], the spectral content of HRV and ECG-derived respiration (EDR) time series from single-lead ECG recordings were analyzed by means of the wavelet transform. The authors proposed a binary SVM for classification (healthy vs. SAHS) and compared its performance with LDA, *k*-NN, and PNN. The proposed SVM classifier reached 100% accuracy in the test set, whereas the PNN showed poor classification performance (80% sensitivity, 50% specificity, and 70% accuracy) probably due to a suboptimal setting of the spread parameter (σ) of the Gaussian function. In a previous study by Khandoker et al. [48], the authors analyzed ECG short-term epochs from nocturnal PSG by means of wavelet decomposition to classify segments into normal breathing, obstructive apnea, and central apnea using a feedforward ANN. The authors reported accuracies of 95.10% in the classification of apneic and normal breathing epochs, 83.40% in the detection of hypopneas, and 98.96% in the classification of obstructive and central apneas. Similarly, Acharya et al. [49] implemented a FFBB ANN using nonlinear measures from the ECG (ApEn, fractal dimension, correlation dimension, largest Lyapunov exponent, and Hurst exponent) to detect apneas, hypopneas, and normal breathing segments. The proposed ANN reached 99.1% accuracy (95.0% sensitivity, 100% specificity), 96.5% accuracy (88.0% sensitivity, 90.0% specificity), and 87.8% accuracy (80.0% sensitivity, 89.5% specificity) in the classification of normal breathing, apneas, and hypopneas, respectively. Lweesky et al. [50] focused on the characterization of the *P*-wave of the ECG in order to feed an ANN aimed at discerning between apnea and normal breathing. The authors reported 90.0% sensitivity, 94.2% specificity, and 92.0% accuracy. In a previous study by Méndez et al. [51], both time and spectral features from the R-to-R interval (RRi) and QRS area time series were used as inputs to a FFBB ANN aimed at discriminating between apneic and nonapneic segments. A sensitivity of 89%, specificity of 86%, and accuracy of 88% were reached in a minute-by-minute classification, whereas 100% accuracy was achieved when the whole recording is classified as normal or apneic. In a recent study, Nguyen et al. [52] proposed a binary ANN to differentiate apnea from normal sleep based on a hear rate complexity measure by means of the recurrence quantification analysis of HRV recordings. In addition, a SVM classifier and an ensemble combining the decisions from both binary classifiers by means of a confidence score (the weighted sum of the output scores of all binary classifiers) were also assessed. The ensemble reached the highest performance (86.37% sensitivity, 83.47% specificity, 85.26% accuracy), whereas single ANN (85.57% sensitivity, 79.09% specificity, 83.23% accuracy) and the SVM (93.72% sensitivity, 65.88% specificity, 84.14% accuracy) classifiers reached slightly lower accuracy but with an unbalanced sensitivity-specificity pair.

ANNs have been also involved in the detection and characterization of snoring and its reliability in SAHS diagnosis. In the study by Fiz et al. [53], a total of 22 features from time and frequency domains (number of snore episodes, average intensity, and power spectral density parameters) were used as inputs to a MLP ANN. A sensitivity of 87% and a specificity of 71%

were achieved using a SAHS cutoff of 5 e/h, whereas 80% sensitivity and 90% specificity were reached for a cutoff of 15 e/h. In a recent study, Nguyen and Won [54] proposed a novel correlational filter ANN (f-MLP) to distinguish normal breathing patterns from snoring patterns during sleep. This ANN implements a correlational filter operation in the frequency domain in a first hidden layer aimed at improving the discriminant power of the spectral content of input patterns, followed by a second feedforward hidden layer. In this study, the authors reported that the f-MLP classifier reached an average accuracy of 96%, outperforming the conventional MLP approach (82% average accuracy).

EEG signals from nocturnal PSG and ANNs have been also used to detect SAHS. Tagluk et al. [55] estimated the quadratic phase coupling of EEG (C3-A2) using bispectral analysis and trained a MLP ANN to detect patients with SAHS. An overall diagnostic accuracy of 96.15% was reached. In the study by Liu et al. [31], both the EEG energy in the theta band and the pupil size were used as inputs to an ANN aimed at discriminating between SAHS patients and healthy subjects. The authors reported 91% overall accuracy in the classification of both groups. Similarly, in the study by Lin et al. [28], the EEG (C3-O1) signal power in the common frequency bands delta, theta, alpha, and beta were estimated by means of the discrete wavelet transform (DWT) and subsequently used to train a FFBB ANN in order to identify SAHS episodes. A sensitivity of 69.64% and a specificity of 44.44% were obtained. The EEG signal has been also used to classify apnea events into obstructive or central. Akşahin et al. computed the synchronization (coherence and mutual information) between EEG channels (C4-A1 and C3-A2) and fed three different ANN-based binary classifiers: conventional FFBB, RBF, and distributed time-delay (DTD) ANNs [56]. The conventional FFBB ANN reached the highest performance in terms of the mean relative absolute error (MRAE = 0.145).

Features from both thoracic and abdominal effort signals have been also used to classify sleep apneas into obstructive, central, and mixed by means of ANNs. In the study by Fontela-Romero et al. [57], the wavelet coefficients from the DWT of the thoracic effort signal feed a Bayesian feedforward ANN, which achieved a mean accuracy of 83.78 ± 1.90%. Similarly, Tagluk et al. [58] analyzed the abdominal respiration signal by means of the wavelet transform and fed a FFBB ANN aimed at classifying apneic events into obstructive, central, and mixed. The proposed methodology achieved an overall accuracy of 78.5% (obstructive: 73.42%; central: 94.23%; mixed: 66.16%). In a recent study by Guijarro-Berdiñas et al. [59], the thoracic effort signal was used to reach the same goal. The DWT was applied to analyze the frequency content of the signal. The wavelet coefficients compose the input patterns of an ensemble of ANNs, which achieved an overall accuracy of 90.27 ± 0.79% (obstructive: 94.62%; central: 95.47%; mixed: 90.45%).

In the study by Weinreich et al. [60], the spectral entropy was used to analyze the frequency content of airflow recordings and feed an ANN trained to discern among SAHS, Cheyne-Stokes respiration, and normal breathing. An overall accuracy of 91.5% was reached in the classification of airflow patterns into obstructive apneas, periodic respiration, and normal breathing during non-REM sleep. Similarly, Várady et al. [61] trained a feedforward ANN to detect apneic events using respiratory signals. Data from both airflow and respiratory inductance plethysmography were used as inputs to the ANN. Up to 93% of input respiratory patterns were correctly classified into normal, apnea, or hypopnea, although no validation was performed.

ANNs have been also used to combine features from different biomedical recordings. In the study by Belal et al. [62], the correlation coefficients between the heart rate (HR), respiratory rate (RR), and SpO_2 signals were computed to detect apnea events in preterm infants in real time. Principal component analysis (PCA) was applied to the correlation coefficients and the components accounting for the 70% of the total variance of the input data fed the MLP ANN, yielding 81.85% sensitivity, 75.83% specificity, and 76.78% accuracy.

It is noteworthy that most studies in the context of SAHS use ANNs for classification purposes, whereas only a few studies apply regression ANNs to estimate the AHI. This is a more challenging task but also a more useful approach, since the AHI is currently a standardized parameter widely used by physicians to assess SAHS severity and to decide whether the CPAP treatment could be effective. In the aforementioned study by El-Solh et al. [19], the authors compared the agreement of two automated regression approaches with the actual AHI from PSG. Multiple linear regression (MLR) and a regression MLP ANN, both trained with anthropometric and clinical variables, were assessed. Significantly higher correlation was reached using the MLP ANN (0.852 vs. 0.509). In the same way, Marcos et al. [63] used spectral and nonlinear features from nocturnal SpO_2 recordings to feed a regression MLP ANN. High intraclass correlation coefficient was reported (ICC = 0.91), which outperformed the conventional MLR approach (ICC = 0.80). Similarly, in a recent study by Gutiérrez-Tobal et al. [25], regression MLP and RBF ANNs were trained to estimate the AHI from PSG using statistical, spectral, and nonlinear features derived from the airflow signal (thermistor). The estimated AHI from the MLP network reached the highest agreement with the PSG-derived AHI (ICC = 0.849 ± 0.002), improving both the RBF and the conventional MLR models.

A snore-based approach has been proposed by de Silva et al. [64] in order to estimate the actual AHI from PSG. Features from the automated analysis of snoring recordings (pitch, first formant, and the quantified recurrence probability density entropy) and the neck circumference were used as inputs to a FFBB ANN to predict the AHI. Averaged 91 ± 6% sensitivity and 89 ± 5% specificity were obtained using a cutoff of 15 e/h for positive SAHS, whereas for a cutoff of 30 e/h, 86 ± 9% sensitivity and 88 ± 5% specificity were achieved. In a similar subsequent study, de Silva et al. [65] proposed this methodology to characterize differences in snoring sounds due to gender and assessed its influence on the performance of a snore-based SAHS screening model. Using an output threshold of 15 e/h, the gender-dependent regression ANN resulted in increased sensitivity (up to 7% higher) and specificity (up to 6% higher) values compared with the gender-neutral model. In the study by Emoto et al. [66], a MLP ANN was used to predict the current value of the breathing sound signal using the preceding samples, i.e., the target output is the current sample, whereas the d-dimensional input feature pattern is composed by the preceding d samples of the breathing signal. In this way, the ANN was applied to distinguish snoring events from normal breathing comparing the network output with an optimized threshold. The proposed method reached an average sensitivity and specificity values of 89.2 and 87.4%, respectively.

3.2. Automated analysis of PSG: sleep staging and sleep/wake automated detection

In order to identify and quantify the number of respiratory events per hour of sleep and derive the AHI, several neuromuscular and cardiorespiratory recordings from the overnight PSG have to be analyzed. However, the interpretation of a PSG is a complex and laborious task even for trained personnel. In this regard, ANNs have demonstrated to be reliable as well as accurate tools to analyze both the macrostructure (automated sleep staging) and the microstructure (transient pattern detection) of sleep [67]. In the context of sleep staging, nonlinear dynamic measures from EEG in combination with pattern classification algorithms have demonstrated to reach clinically significant results in sleep disorders diagnosis, treatment monitoring, and drug efficacy assessment [68]. In fact, a number of automated algorithms are currently implemented into commercialized software tools for PSG analysis. Nevertheless, the performance of automated pattern recognition algorithms varies greatly depending on the number of stages involved in the classification task, from 2 (wake vs. sleep) to 5 (wake, REM, N1-N3) states (6 classes if the conventional Rechtschaffen and Kales classification is used). In addition, the accuracy is also influenced by the number and kind of recordings involved in the classification task (EEG, EOG, and/or EMG). **Table 2** summarizes the main characteristics of significant studies focused on applications of ANNs for automated sleep staging, arousal quantification, and drowsiness detection.

In the study by Becq et al. [69], the relative power in the common frequency bands of the EEG (C3-A2), as well as the overall variance of EEG and EMG signals, was used to feed a 6-class MLP ANN. The proposed method reached the same performance as a *k*-NN classifier, achieving 28 ± 2% error rate. Ventouras et al. [70] trained a MLP ANN to detect sleep spindles using a bandpass filtered EEG channel (Cz) without feature extraction. The classifier achieved 80.2% sensitivity and 95.0% specificity in the whole sleep record after a consensus agreement among independent scorers. In the study by Caffarel et al. [71], an ANN-based commercial software using a single-channel EEG (Cz-A1) was assessed. The overall agreement between automated and manual scoring was relatively low in a 4-class classification task (*kappa* = 0.305) and slightly better in a 2-class classification task (*kappa* = 0.449). In a later study by Ebrahimi et al. [72], wavelet decomposition and ANNs were used to perform 4-class sleep staging using the EEG signal. An overall sensitivity of 84.2 ± 3.9%, specificity of 94.4 ± 4.5%, and accuracy of 93.0 ± 4.0% were reported. Wavelet coefficients from the EEG (P3-P4) and a backpropagation ANN were also used in the study carried out by Sinha [73]. The author reported accuracies of 96.84%, 93.68%, and 95.52% in the detection of sleep spindles, REM sleep, and awake state, respectively. More recently, Hsu et al. [32] computed energy-based measures from a single EEG channel (Fpz-Cz) to feed a recurrent neural classifier (RNN), which achieved an overall accuracy of 87.2% in a 5-class classification task.

Adding features from additional biomedical signals as inputs to the ANN does not seem to improve significantly the classification performance. In the study by Shambroom et al. [74], a commercial wireless device for automated sleep staging based on the combined activity of EEG, EOG, and EMG is assessed. The Zeo device implements an ANN that achieved 81.1% agreement for light sleep versus deep sleep classification and 93.6% agreement for sleep versus wake classification when the gold standard is a consensus between two independent

Author (year) [Ref.]	ANN model	Purpose	Target function/ class(es)	Input variables	Performance metrics
Becq et al. (2005) [69]	MLP	6-class classification	Wake/NREM 1-4/ REM	EEG (C3-A2) (overall variance, relative power) EMG (overall variance)	ER: 28 ± 2%
Ventouras et al. (2005) [70]	MLP	Binary classification	Sleep spindle detection	Single channel EEG (Cz)	80.2% Se, 95.0% Sp
Caffarel et al. (2006) [71]	NS	4-class 2-class	Wake/light sleep/ deep sleep/REM Wake vs. sleep	EEG (Cz-A1)	$k = 0.305$ $k = 0.449$
Ebrahimi et al. (2008) [72]	NS	4-class classification	Wake/ NREM1+REM/ NREM2/SWS	Wavelet decomposition of single channel EEG	84.2% Se, 94.4% Sp, 93.0% Acc
Sinha (2008) [73]	FFBB	3-class classification	Sleep spindles (SS)/REM/Awake	Wavelet coefficients from EEG	95.35% Acc (overall) 96.84% Acc (SS) 93.68% Acc (REM) 95.52% Acc (Awake)
Hsu et al. (2013) [32]	RNN FFBB PNN	5-class classification	Wake/NREM1/ NREM2/SWS/ REM	Energy features from single-channel EEG	87.2% overall Acc 81.1% overall Acc 81.8% overall Acc
Shambroom et al. (2012) [74]	NS	Binary classification	Sleep *vs.* wake Light *vs.* deed sleep	Combined EEG/EOG/ EMG activity by a single lead (wireless Zeo)	93.6% Acc 81.1% Acc
Griessenberger et al. (2013) [75]	NS	Classification (4-class)	Wake/REM/light sleep/deep sleep	Combined EEG/ EOG/EMG activity by a single lead (wireless Zeo)	72.6% overall Acc
Tagluk et al. (2010) [76]	FFBB	Classification (5-class)	NREM 1 to 4/ REM	Filtered EOG and EMG	74.7% overall Acc 72.6% Acc (NREM1) 73.3% Acc (NREM2) 78.0% Acc (NREM3) 72.3% Acc (NREM4) 77.3% Acc (REM)
Chapotot and Becq (2009) [77]	Ensemble MLP	Classification (6-class)	Wake/N1 to N3/ REM/Movement	Statistical, spectral, nonlinear features from EEG and EMG	36 ± 15% error rate 0.48 ± 0.18 k 34% Acc (Wake) 43% Acc (N1) 51% Acc (N2) 82% Acc (N3) 82% Acc (REM) 13% Acc (Mov.)
Charbonnier et al. (2011) [78]	Ensemble MLP	Classification (5-class)	Wake/NREM1/ NREM2/SWS/ REM	Time and spectral (Fourier analysis) features from EEG, EMG, and EOG	85.5% overall Acc 78.1% Acc (Wake) 64.8% Acc (NREM1) 86.9% Acc (NREM2) 94.8% Acc (SWS) 79.3% Acc (REM)

Author (year) [Ref.]	ANN model	Purpose	Target function/ class(es)	Input variables	Performance metrics
Álvarez-Estevez and Moret-Bonillo (2009) [79]	FLD QD SVM FFBB	Classification (binary)	Arousal detection	Energy in common bands of EEG (Fourier analysis)	0.196 ± 0.015 ER 0.195 ± 0.015 ER 0.140 ± 0.012 ER 0.092 ± 0.010 ER
Patel et al. (2011) [85]	FFBB	Classification (binary)	Alert *vs.* fatigue	Spectral power (Fourier analysis) of HRV	90% Acc
Lin et al. (2006) [86]	FNN	Regression	Driver's drowsiness level estimation	Spectral power of EEG and ICA	Pearson correlation: 0.913 ± 0.027
Kurt et al. (2009) [87]	MLP	Classification (3-class)	Awake/drowsy/ sleep	Wavelet decomposition of EEG, EOG and chin-EMG	97–98% overall Acc
Garcés et al. (2014) [88]	FFBB	Classification (binary)	Alert *vs.* drowsiness	Time, spectral, and wavelet decomposition of single-lead EEG	87.4% Se, 83.6% Sp

Notes: ER: error rate; Se: sensitivity; Sp: specificity; *k*: *kappa* coefficient of classification ability; Acc: accuracy; NS: not specified; MLP: multilayer perceptron; SWS: slow wave sleep; FFBB: feed-forward back-propagation; SS: sleep spindles; RNN: recurrent ANN; PNN: probabilistic neural network; FLD: Fisher's linear discriminant; QD: quadratic discriminant; SVM: support vector machine; FNN: fuzzy ANN; ICA: independent component analysis.

Table 2. Performance and the most relevant characteristics of the studies using ANNs in the context of sleep staging, arousal detection, and drowsiness monitoring.

expert scorers. In a subsequent similar study [75], the same wireless system achieved an overall agreement of 72.6% in a 4-class approach (Wake, REM, light, and deep sleep). Tagluk et al. [76] used bandpass filtered EOG and EMG recordings as inputs to a feedforward ANN in a 5-class classification task, achieving an overall accuracy of 74.7 ± 1.63%. Similarly, using statistical, spectral, and nonlinear features from EEG and EMG signals and an ensemble classifier based on multiple MLP ANNs, 64% overall performance was achieved for wakefulness, movement, and intermediate sleep detection, while 82% accuracy was reached for deep and paradoxical sleep detection [77]. In the study carried out by Charbonnier et al. [78], 85.5% overall accuracy was reached using EEG-, EOG-, and EMG-derived features as inputs to an ensemble of 4 MLP ANN for 5-class automated sleep staging.

In the study by Álvarez-Estevez and Moret-Bonillo [79], two EEG channels (C2-A2 and C4-A1) and the submental EMG channel were analyzed to automatically detect arousals in the context of SAHS classification. For these signals, the energy in the conventional frequency bands was computed by means of the Fourier transform and four automated expert systems were trained: Fisher's linear and quadratic discriminants, a SVM, and a feedforward ANN. The ANN reached the highest performance, achieving 92% accuracy and 0.0921 ± 0.0098 error rate.

Besides ANNs, it is noteworthy that several competing algorithms have been applied for automated sleep staging, such as Gaussian mixture models (88.4% overall accuracy, 6-class,

EEG-based) [80], discrete hidden Markov models (85.29% overall accuracy, 5-class, EEG/EOG/EMG-based) [81], linear (73.7% overall accuracy, 4-class, HRV-based), and quadratic (63.7% overall accuracy, 4-class, HRV-based) discriminant analysis (81% accuracy, 5-class, EEG/EOG/EMG/ECG-based) [82, 83], SVM (89.39% accuracy 5-class, single EEG) [84], DTs (72.6% accuracy, 5-class, EEG/EOG single lead). In the same way as ANNs, these approaches are characterized by variable performance.

3.2.1. Driver's drowsiness detection

A relevant application of ANNs in the context of SAHS is the detection of drivers' fatigue and/or drowsiness, which is an important issue for patients suffering from SBD. In this regard, different physiological signals have been used to monitor alertness, such as spectral analysis of HRV (90% accuracy) [85] and EEG (0.913 ± 0.027 correlation between actual and estimated alertness levels) [86], wavelet coefficients of EEG combined with features from EOG and EMG (97–98% 3-class overall accuracy) [87], and time, spectral, and wavelet features from single-lead EEG [88]. Neuromuscular (EEG, EOG, EMG) and cardiac (ECG) signals have been analyzed predominantly in order to detect drowsiness, though additional physiological recordings (oximetry, skin conductance), physical measures (eye movement/blinks, face and mouth images), and driver's performance measures (steering wheel movements) have been also proposed as inputs to different pattern recognition methods, specially Bayesian networks, SVMs, and ensembles of linear classifiers [89–91]. The main limitation of these automated algorithms is that a great amount of data is needed to perform an accurate training of the pattern recognition method. Nonetheless, alertness monitoring systems are already incorporated in many high-end vehicles.

3.3. Neural networks and continuous positive airway pressure

The incorporation of automated decision support systems in the common clinical practice of SAHS diagnosis is still very limited. Conversely, the implementation of artificial intelligence-based expert systems in treatment devices for sleep-related breathing disorders therapy increased significantly during the last decade. In this regard, the exponential technological development of continuous positive airway pressure (CPAP) devices relies on the automated analysis of breathing patterns by means of expert systems, most of them based on ANNs. Currently, CPAP is the primary preferred treatment of mild, moderate, and severe SAHS and thus it is considered the standard of care. During CPAP treatment, a continuous pressure of air is delivered to the patient's upper airway to keep patency [92]. Though nonintrusive, simple, and effective, the device delivers an unnecessary constant high pressure during the whole night whatever the actual patient's needs, which decreases comfort and in turn treatment compliance. This is the main limitation of CPAP and thus the most relevant improvements during the last years focused on the modulation of the pressure delivered by the device in order to fit patient's needs. In this regard, the major companies operating in the SAHS therapy market incorporated to their devices automated algorithms to monitor and modulate the breathing gas pressure. Nevertheless, most manufactures provide no technical data about the design and implementation of their automated signal processing algorithms and thus they are blackboxes hard to interpret and assess.

http://dx.doi.org/10.5772/66570

As aforementioned, determining the optimal therapeutic pressure has been a major goal of research regarding CPAP treatment. Different respiratory-related signals have been assessed for automated regulation of the pressure. Airflow, SpO_2 from oximetry, HRV, pharyngeal wall vibration, and snoring sounds have been involved in automated algorithms aimed at detecting airflow limitation and respiratory events. Among them, the analysis of the airflow profile is the most widely used method [93, 94]. In this regard, several algorithms have been patented during the last years, which reflect the increasing interest of leading companies in this field. In the patent by Norman et al. [93], a pretrained ANN fed with shape-based features from the airflow signal is used to detect the presence of airflow limitation in each individual patient's breath. Eklund et al. [95] granted a patent for automatically adjusting the flow pressure when respiratory events are detected. To achieve this goal, an ANN is fed with respiration-related variables. In a recent granted patent, Waxman et al. [96] proposed a Large Memory Storage and Retrieval (LAMSTAR) neural network to process patient's physiological data in order to predict breathing events and control the airway pressure level supplied to the user. This algorithm reached high prediction ability within the 30 s preceding the respiratory event [96]. Similarly, in the patent by Hedner et al. [97], the authors describe a pattern recognition system based on a plurality of ANNs aimed at controlling the therapy breathing support in order to increase its effectiveness. Leading companies, such as Philips Respironics, ResMed, or Fisher & Paykel, incorporated these algorithms into their CPAP devices. Nevertheless, additional research is still needed to further assess whether these technological advances can effectively improve CPAP adherence.

Automatic detection of wake and sleep states is a novel approach for enhancing patient's comfort [98, 99]. In the study carried out by Ayappa et al. [98], the authors proposed an ANN to detect irregular respiration characteristics of sleep/wake transitions. In this study, the CPAP flow signal is parameterized by means of breath timing and amplitude measures, which subsequently feed the ANN in order to detect irregular breathing. This algorithm is used in the commercial system SensAwake™ (Fisher & Paykel, Auckland, NZ) in order to automatically decrease the therapeutic pressure when the patient is awake [99]. This ANN has demonstrated to be effective for sleep onset and awakening detection, though there is still little if any evidence supporting its actual long-term influence on patient's comfort and CPAP compliance.

In order to obtain the optimal CPAP pressure level for a patient, an individual titration procedure is needed. This technique is aimed at estimating the continuous pressure that normalizes the patient's sleep and breathing during in-lab PSG, which contributes to increase the large waiting lists. Therefore, alternative methods are demanded. In this regard, El-Solh et al. [100] designed and trained a GRNN aimed at estimating the most effective continuous pressure using demographic and anthropometric variables (those from the Hoffstein formula, i.e., age, gender, BMI, neck circumference, and AHI). The authors reported high agreement between the optimal pressure determined by standard titration during overnight PSG and the pressure predicted by the ANN. In a later randomized study, El-Solh et al. [101] reported that this ANN can be effectively used to guide CPAP titration. The authors showed that automated titration procedures using this methodology reached the optimal CPAP pressure at a shorter time interval compared to conventional PSG-based titration, as well as lower titration failure.

4. Conclusion

Researchers carried out an exhaustive study during the last decades focused on the design of automated expert systems derived from artificial intelligence able to help physicians in their daily practice. Accordingly, several computer-aided decision support systems have been proposed to overcome limitations of the standard diagnostic methodology for SAHS. Among all the automated prediction methods, ANNs are probably the most widely used pattern recognition algorithm in the context of SAHS management. Their flexibility to model complex nonlinear problems and their higher generalization ability allow ANNs to reach higher performance rates both in classification and regression problems. In this regard, several applications of ANNs have been developed, such as classification of patients suspected of suffering from SAHS, AHI estimation, detection and quantification of respiratory events, apneic events classification, automated sleep staging and arousal detection, alertness monitoring systems, and airflow pressure optimization in PAP-based devices. On the other hand, the most common limitation of ANNs relates to the interpretation of the results in terms of the significance of the variables involved in the model. In this way, ANNs are most times viewed as blackboxes that are not able to generate understandable rules, which is the main weakness of neural-based classifiers. Conversely, both decision trees and probabilistic networks also reach high performance by providing interpretable rules and relationships between input variables.

Regarding input features, ANNs are able to deal with high-dimensional spaces composed of several features. This is especially useful when working with a lot of data sources providing information about the problem under study, such as symptoms reported by the patient, physical examination, sleep questionnaires, or PSG, among others. However, it is important to highlight that, sometimes, researchers try to compose a wide initial feature set in order to gather as much information as possible, including features from signal processing algorithms regardless of their relevance or clinical meaning. In this way, feature selection strategies are very useful to distinguish the more significant ones. In addition, dimensionality reduction algorithms allow ANNs to deal with the curse of dimensionality problem and to control overfitting. Nevertheless, just a few studies apply feature selection techniques before the classification stage.

ANNs have yielded reliable and accurate applications in the context of SAHS detection. Nevertheless, it is noteworthy that, in the last years, there is a trend to use different pattern recognition algorithms, particularly SVMs and ensemble classifiers. SVMs have emerged as powerful tools able to achieve significantly high performance both in classification and regression problems. They are kernel-based maximum margin classifiers, i.e., the decision boundary is determined by a subset of the training data samples in a transformed space in which the margin (the distance between the boundary and the closest samples) is maximized. In this way, the optimization problem is relatively straightforward [18]. Several recent studies have demonstrated the usefulness of SVMs in the framework of SAHS management [102–105]. Moreover, in the present research, some studies were reviewed reporting that SVM-based classifiers reached higher accuracy than ANNs [23, 45, 52]. Unlike ANNs, SVMs are capable to minimize both structural and empirical risk, leading to higher generalization ability even when working with limited training datasets [103]. On the other hand, they are also characterized as blackboxes and usually higher computational time is needed to optimize the classifier [27]. Unfortunately, there are few studies assessing the performance of different classification approaches in the same conditions (population under study and equal optimization of input parameters), leading to biased results and poor generalization. Open access databases, such as the *Physionet* or the *Sleep Heart Health Study* (SHHS), provide a common benchmark to properly assess the performance of different methodologies using the same data. Nevertheless, these databases are limited and most studies are carried out using no publicly available datasets, which restricts comparisons.

In addition, it is also noteworthy that ensemble classifiers, from the simplest majority vote to the more complex bagging, boosting, and stacking algorithms, have been recently introduced in the context of SAHS in order to improve classification performance [106, 107]. It is obvious that misclassified samples are not always the same when using different classification algorithms. Accordingly, improved performance may be reached when working with several classifiers at the same time. In this way, ensemble algorithms take advantage of the information provided by all the classifiers involved in the classification or regression task. The studies by Guijarro-Berdiñas et al. [59] and Nguyen et al. [52] demonstrated the reliability and efficacy of ANN-based ensembles. Nevertheless, further research is still need in order to exploit the full potential of this approach in the context of SAHS diagnosis.

Acknowledgements

This research has been partially supported by projects 153/2015 and 158/2015 of the Sociedad Española de Neumología y Cirugía Torácica (SEPAR), the project RTC-2015-3446-1 from the Ministerio de Economía y Competitividad and the European Regional Development Fund (FEDER), and the project VA037U16 from the Consejería de Educación de la Junta de Castilla y León and FEDER. D. Álvarez was in receipt of a Juan de la Cierva grant from the Ministerio de Economía y Competitividad.

Author details

Daniel Álvarez[1, 2], Ana Cerezo-Hernández[1], Graciela López-Muñiz[1], Tania Álvaro-De Castro[1], Tomás Ruiz-Albi[1], Roberto Hornero[2] and Félix del Campo[1, 2]*

*Address all correspondence to: fsas@telefonica.net

1 Sleep-Ventilation Unit, Pneumology Service, Río Hortega University Hospital, Valladolid, Spain

2 Biomedical Engineering Group, University of Valladolid, Valladolid, Spain

References

[1] Lisboa PJ, Taktak AFG. The use of artificial neural network in decision supports in cancer. A systematic review. Neural Networks. 2006;19:408–415. DOI: 10.1016/j.neunet.2005.10.007

[2] Adams ST, Leveson SH. Clinical prediction rules. BMJ. 2012;**344**:d8312–d8312. DOI: 10.1136/bmj.d8312

[3] Marcos JV, Hornero R, Álvarez D, Del Campo F, Aboy M. Automated detection of obstructive sleep apnoea syndrome from oxygen saturation recordings using linear discriminant analysis. Medical & Biological Engineering & Computing. 2010;**48**:895–902. DOI: 10.1007/s11517-010-0646-6

[4] Álvarez D, Hornero R, Marcos JV, Del Campo F. Feature selection from nocturnal oximetry using genetic algorithms to assist in obstructive sleep apnoea diagnosis. Medical Engineering & Physics. 2012;**34**:1049–1057. DOI: 10.1016/j.medengphy.2011.11.009

[5] Pandey B, Mishra RB. Knowledge and intelligent computing system in medicine. Computers in Biology and Medicine. 2009;**39**:215-30. DOI: 10.1016/j.compbiomed.2008.12.008

[6] Raudys S. Statistical and neural classifiers. An integrated approach to design. London: Springer; 2001. ISBN: 1-85233-297-2

[7] McCulloch WS, Pitts W. A logical calculus of the ideas immanent in nervous activity. Bulletin of Mathematical Biophysics. 1943;**5**:115. DOI:10.1007/BF02478259

[8] Flemons WW, Littner MR, Rowlet JA, Gay P, Anderson WM, Hudgel DW, McEvoy RD, Loube DI. Home diagnosis of sleep apnea: A systematic review of the literature. Chest. 2003;**124**:1543–1579. DOI: 10.1378/chest.124.4.1543

[9] Qaseem A, Dallas P, Owens DK, Starkey M, Holty J-EC, Shekelle P. Diagnosis of obstructive sleep apnea in adults: A clinical practice guideline from the American College of Physicians. Annals of Internal Medicine. 2014;**161**:210–220. DOI: 10.7326/M12-3187

[10] Álvarez-Estevez D, Moret-Bonillo V. Computer-assisted diagnosis of the sleep apnea-hypopnea syndrome: a review. Sleep Disorders. 2015;**2015**:1–33. DOI: 10.1155/2015/237878

[11] Kocak O, Bayrak T, Erdamar A, Ozparlak L, Telatar Z, Erogul O. Automated detection and classification of sleep apnea types using electrocardiogram (ECG) and electroencephalogram (EEG) features. Advances in Electrocardiograms – Clinical Applications, PhD. Richard Millis (Ed.). Croatia: InTech; 2012. ISBN: 978-953-307-902-8.

[12] Álvarez D, Gutiérrez-Tobal GC, Del Campo F, Hornero R. Positive airway pressure and electrical stimulation methods for obstructive sleep apnea treatment: a patent review (2005–2014). Expert Opinion on Therapeutic Patents. 2015;**25**:971–989. DOI: 10.1517/13543776.2015.1054094

[13] Haykin S. Neural networks: A comprehensive foundation. New Jersey: Prentice Hall Inc; 1999.

[14] Rojas R. Neural networks. A systematic introduction. Berlin Heidelberg: Springer Verlag; 1996. DOI: 10.1007/978-3-642-61068-4

[15] Zhang GP. Neural networks for classification: a survey. IEEE Transactions on Systems, Man and Cibernetics, Part C. 2000;**30;**451–462. DOI: 10.1109/5326.897072

[16] Hush DR, Horne BG. Progress in supervised neural networks. IEEE Signal Processing Magazine. 1993;**10:**8–39. DOI: 10.1109/79.180705

[17] Bishop CM. Neural networks for pattern recognition. New York: Oxford University Press; 1995. ISBN: 0-19-853864

[18] Bishop CM. Pattern recognition and machine learning. New York: Springer; 2006. ISBN: 0-387-31073-8

[19] El-Solh AA, Mador MJ, Ten-Brock E, Shucard DW, Abul-Khoudoud M, Grant BJ. Validity of neural network in sleep apnea. Sleep. 1999;**22**:105–111.

[20] Marcos JV, Hornero R, Álvarez D, Del Campo F, Zamarrón C, López M. Utility of multilayer perceptron neural network classifiers in the diagnosis of the obstructive sleep apnoea syndrome from nocturnal oximetry. Computer Methods and Programs in Biomedicine. 2008;**92**:79–89. DOI: 10.1016/j.cmpb.2008.05.006

[21] Karamanli H, Yalcinoz T, Yalcinoz MA, Yalcinoz T. A prediction model based on artificial neural networks for the diagnosis of obstructive sleep apnea. Sleep Breath. 2016;**20**:509–514. DOI 10.1007/s11325-015-1218-7

[22] Marcos JV, Hornero R, Álvarez D, Nabney IT, Del Campo F, Zamarrón C. The classification of oximetry signals using Bayesian neural networks to assist in the detection of obstructive sleep apnoea syndrome. Physiological Measurement. 2010;**31**:375–394. DOI: doi:10.1088/0967-3334/31/3/007

[23] Khandoker AH, Karmakar CHK, Palaniswami M. Automated recognition of patients with obstructive sleep apnoea using wavelet-based features of electrocardiogram recordings. Computers in Biology and Medicine. 2009;**39**:88–96. DOI: 10.1016/j.compbiomed.2008.11.003

[24] Marcos JV, Hornero R, Álvarez D, Del Campo F, López M, Zamarrón C. Radial basis function classifiers to help in the diagnosis of the obstructive sleep apnoea syndrome from nocturnal oximetry. Medical & Biological Engineering & Computing. 2008;**46**:323–332. DOI: 10.1007/s11517-007-0280-0

[25] Gutiérrez-Tobal GC, Álvarez D, Marcos JV, Del Campo F, Hornero R. Pattern recognition in airflow recordings to assist in the sleep apnoea–hypopnoea syndrome diagnosis. Medical & Biological Engineering & Computing. 2013;**51**:1367–1380. DOI 10.1007/s11517-013-1109-7

[26] Huang S-H, Teng N-C, Wang K-J, Chen K-H, Lee H-C, Wang P-C. Use of oximetry as a screening tool for obstructive sleep apnea: a case study in Taiwan. Journal of Medical Systems. 2015;**39**:29. DOI 10.1007/s10916-015-0195-5

[27] Wang K-J, Chen K-H, Huang S-H, Teng N-C. A prognosis tool based on fuzzy anthropometric and questionnaire data for obstructive sleep apnea. Journal of Medical Systems. 2016;**40**:110. DOI: 10.1007/s10916-016-0464-y

[28] Lin R, Lee R-G, Tseng C-L, Zhou H-K, Chao C-F, Jiang J-A. A new approach for identifying sleep apnea syndrome using wavelet transform and neural networks. Biomedical Engineering: Applications, Basis and Communications. 2006;**18**:138–143. DOI: 10.4015/S1016237206000233

[29] Polat K, Yosunkaya S, Güneş S. Comparison of different classifier algorithms on the automated detection of obstructive sleep apnea syndrome. Journal of Medical Systems. 2008;**32**:243–250. DOI 10.1007/s10916-008-9129-9

[30] Ghandeharioun H, Rezaeitalab F, Lotfi R. Accurate estimation of obstructive sleep apnea severity using non-polysomnographic features for home-based screening. Iranian Journal of Public Health. 2015;**44:**1433–1435.

[31] Liu D, Pang Z, Lloyd SR. A neural network method for detection of obstructive sleep apnea and narcolepsy based on pupil size and EEG. IEEE Transactions on Neural Networks. 2008;**19:**308–318. DOI: 10.1109/TNN.2007.908634

[32] Hsu Y-L, Yang Y-T, Wang J-S, Hsu C-Y. Automatic sleep stage recurrent neural classifier using energy features of EEG signals. Neurocomputing. 2013;**104:**105–114. DOI: 10.1016/j.neucom.2012.11.003

[33] Hornik K. Approximation capabilities of multilayer feedforward networks. Neural Networks. 1991;**4:**251–257. DOI: 10.1016/0893-6080(91)90009-T

[34] Basheer IA, Hajmeer M. Artificial neural networks: fundamentals, computing, design, and application. Journal of Microbiological Methods. 2000;**43**:3–31. DOI: 10.1016/S0167-7012(00)00201-3

[35] Sethi IK, Jain AK. Artificial neural networks and statistical pattern recognition. Machine intelligence and pattern recognition series, VOL. II. Amsterdam: Elsevier; 1991. ISBN: 0-444-88740-7

[36] Jain AK, Duin RPW, Mao J. Statistical pattern recognition: a review. IEEE Transactions on Pattern Analysis and Machine Intelligence. 2000;**22;**4–37. DOI: 10.1109/34.824819

[37] Foster KR, Koprowski R, Skufca JD. Machine learning, medical diagnosis, and biomedical engineering research – commentary. BioMedical Engineering OnLine. 2014;**13**:94. DOI: 10.1186/1475-925X-13-94

[38] Dayhoff JE, Deleo JM. Artificial neural networks: opening the black box. Cancer. 2001;**91**:1615–1635.

[39] Graupe D. Principles of artificial neural networks. 3rd edition. Singapore: World Scientific Publishing Co.; 2007. ISBN: 978-981-4522-73-1

[40] Baxt WG. Application of artificial neural networks to clinical medicine. Lancet. 1995;**346**:1135–1138.

[41] Siristatidis CS, Chrelias C, Pouliakis A, Katsimanis E, Kassanos D. Artificial neural networks in gynaecological diseases: current and potential future applications. Medical Science Monitor. 2010;**16**:RA231-6.

[42] Amato F, López A, Peña-Méndez EM, Vaňhara P, Hampl A, Havel J. Artificial neural networks in medical diagnosis. Journal of Applied Biomedicine. 2013;**11**:47–58. DOI:10.2478/v10136-012-0031-x

[43] Kirby SD, Danter W, George CFP, Francovic T, Ruby RRF, Ferguson KA. Neural network prediction of obstructive sleep apnea from clinical criteria. Chest. 1999;**116**:409–415. DOI: 10.1378/chest.116.2.409

[44] De Chazal P, Heneghan C, McNicholas WT. Multimodal detection of sleep apnoea using electrocardiogram and oximetry signals. Philosophical Transactions of the Royal Society A. 2009;**367**:369–389. DOI: 10.1098/rsta.2008.0156

[45] Su CT, Chen KH, Chen LF, Wang PC, Hsiao YH. Prediagnosis of obstructive sleep apnea via multiclass MTS. Computational and Mathematical Methods in Medicine. 2012;**2012**:212498. DOI: 10.1155/2012/212498

[46] Almazaydeh L, Faezipour M, Elleithy K. A, editors. Neural network system for detection of obstructive sleep apnea through SpO_2 signal features. International Journal of Advanced Computer Science and Applications. 2012;**3**:7–11. ISBN: 2156-5570

[47] Sánchez-Morillo D, Gross N. Probabilistic neural network approach for the detection of SAHS from overnight pulse oximetry. Medical & Biological Engineering & Computing. 2013;**51**:305. DOI 10.1007/s11517-012-0995-4

[48] Khandoker AH, Gubbi J, Palaniswami M. Recognizing central and obstructive sleep apnea events from normal breathing events in ECG recordings. Computers in Cardiology. 2008;**35**:681–684. DOI: 10.1109/CIC.2008.4749133

[49] Acharya UR, Chua ECP, Faust O, Lim TC, Lim LFB. Automated detection of sleep apnea from electrocardiogram signals using nonlinear parameters. Physiological Measurement. 2011;**32**:287–303. DOI: 10.1088/0967-3334/32/3/002

[50] Lweesy K, Fraiwan L, Khasawnch N, Dickhuash. New automated detection method of OSA based on artificial neural networks using P wave shape and time changes. Journal of Medical Systems. 2011;**35**:723–734. DOI: DOI 10.1007/s10916-009-9409-z

[51] Méndez MO, Bianchi AM, Matteucci M, Cerutti S, Penzel T. Sleep apnea screening by autoregressive models from a single ECG lead. IEEE Transactions on Biomedical Engineering. 2009;**56**:2838–2850. DOI: 10.1109/TBME.2009.2029563

[52] Nguyen HD, Wilkins BA, Cheng Q, Benjamin BA. An online sleep apnea detection method based on recurrence quantification analysis. IEEE Journal of Biomedical and Health Informatics. 2014;**18**:1285–1293] DOI: 10.1109/JBHI.2013.2292928

[53] Fiz JA, Jané R, Solá-Soler J, Abad J, García M, Morera J. Continuous analysis and monitoring of snores and their relationship to the apnea-hypopnea index. Laryngoscope. 2010;**120**:854–862. DOI: 10.1002/lary.20815

[54] Nguyen TL, Won Y. Sleep snoring detection using multi-layer neural networks. Bio-Medical Materials and Engineering. 2015;**26:**S1749–S1755. DOI: 10.3233/BME-151475

[55] Tagluk ME, Segzin N. A new approach for estimation of obstructive sleep apnea syndrome. Expert Systems with Applications. 2011;**38**:5346–5351. DOI: 10.1016/j.eswa.2010.10.022

[56] Akşahin M, Aydın S, Fırat H, Eroğul O. Artificial apnea classification with quantitative sleep EEG synchronization. Journal of Medical Systems 2012;**36**(1):139–144. DOI: 10.1007/s10916-010-9453-8

[57] Fontenla-Romero O, Guijarro-Berdiñas B, Alonso-Betanzos A, Moret-Bonillo V. A new method for sleep apnea classification using wavelets and feedforward neural networks. Artificial Intelligence in Medicine. 2005;**34**:65–76. DOI: 10.1016/j.artmed.2004.07.014

[58] Tagluk ME, Akin M, Sezgin N. Classıfıcation of sleep apnea by using wavelet transform and artificial neural networks. Expert Systems with Applications. 2010;**37**:1600–1607. DOI:

[59] Guijarro-Berdiñas B, Hernández-Pereira E, Peteiro-Barral D. A mixture of experts for classifying sleep apneas. Expert Systems with Applications. 2012;**39:**7084–7092. DOI: 10.1016/j.eswa.2012.01.037

[60] Weinreich G, Armitstead J, Teschler H. Pattern recognition of obstructive sleep apnoea and Cheyne–Stokes respiration. Physiological Measurement. 2008;**29**:869. DOI: 10.1088/0967-3334/29/8/002

[61] Várady P, Micsik T, Benedek S, Benyó Z. A novel method for the detection of apnea and hypopnea events in respiration signals. IEEE Transactions on Biomedical Engineering. 2002;**49**:936–942. DOI: 10.1109/TBME.2002.802009

[62] Belal SY, Emmerson AJ, Beatty PC. Automatic detection of apnoea of prematurity. Physiological Measurement. 2011;**32**(5):523–542. DOI: 10.1088/0967-3334/32/5/003

[63] Marcos JV, Hornero R, Álvarez D, Aboy M, Del Campo F. Automated prediction of the apnea-hypopnea index from nocturnal oximetry recordings. IEEE Transactions on Biomedical Engineering. 2012;**59**:141–149. DOI: 10.1109/TBME.2011.2167971

[64] de Silva S, Abeyratne UR, Hukins C. A method to screen obstructive sleep apnea using multi-variable non-intrusive measurements. Physiological Measurement. 2011;**32**(4):445–465. DOI: 10.1088/0967-3334/32/4/006

[65] de Silva S, Abeyratne UR, Hukins C. Impact of gender on snore-based obstructive sleep apnea screening. Physiological Measurement. 2012;**33**:587. DOI: 10.1088/0967-3334/33/4/587

[66] Emoto T, Abeyratne UR, Chen Y, Kawata I, Akutagawa M, Kinouchi Y. Artificial neural networks for breathing and snoring episode detection in sleep sounds. Physiological Measurement. 2012;**33**(10):1675–1689. DOI: 10.1088/0967-3334/33/10/1675

[67] Motamedi-Fakhr S, Moshrefi-Torbati M, Hill M, Hill CM, White PR. Signal processing techniques applied to human sleep EEG signals—A review. Biomedical Signal Processing and Control. 2014;**10**:21–33. DOI: 10.1016/j.bspc.2013.12.003

[68] Acharya UR, Bhat S, Faust O, Adeli H, Chua EC-P, Lim WJE, Koh JEW. Nonlinear dynamics measures for automated EEG-based sleep stage detection. European Neurology. 2015;**74**:268–287. DOI: 10.1159/000441975

[69] Becq G, Charbonnier S, Chapotot F, Buguet A, Bourdon L, Baconnier P. Comparison between five classifiers for automatic scoring of human sleep recordings. Studies in Computational Intelligence (SCI) Vol. 4. Berlin, Heidelberg: Springer-Verlag; 2005. pp. 113–127. DOI: DOI: 10.1007/11011620_8

[70] Ventouras EM, Monoyiou EA, Ktonas PY, Paparrigopoulos T, Dikeos DG, Uzunoglu NK, Soldatos CR. Sleep spindle detection using artificial neural networks trained with filtered time-domain EEG: A feasibility study. Computer Methods and Programs in Biomedicine. 2005;**78**:191–207. DOI: 10.1016/j.cmpb.2005.02.006

[71] Caffarel J, Gibson GJ, Harrison JP, Griffiths CJ, Drinnan MJ. Comparison of manual sleep staging with automated neural network-based analysis in clinical practice. Medical & Biological Engineering & Computing. 2006;**44**:105–110. DOI: 10.1007/s11517-005-0002-4

[72] Ebrahimi F, Mikaeili M, Estrada E, Nazeran H. Automatic sleep stage classification based on EEG signals by using neural networks and wavelet packet coefficients. In: Proceedings of the 30th Annual International Conference of the IEEE Engineering in Medicine and Biology Society; 20–25 August 2008; Vacouver. New York: IEEE; 2008. pp. 1151–1154. DOI: 10.1109/IEMBS.2008.4649365

[73] Sinha RK. Artificial neural network and wavelet based automated detection of sleep spindles, REM sleep and wake states. Journal of Medical Systems. 2008;**32**:291–299. DOI: 10.1007/s10916-008-9134-z

[74] Shambroom JR, Fábregas SE, Johnstone J. Validation of an automated wireless system to monitor sleep in healthy adults. Journal of Sleep Research. 2012;**21**:221–230. DOI: 10.1111/j.1365-2869.2011.00944.x

[75] Griessenberger H, Heib DPJ, Kunz AB, Hoedlmoser K, Schabus M. Assessment of a wireless headband for automatic sleep scoring. Sleep Breath. 2013;**17**:747–752. DOI 10.1007/s11325-012-0757-4

[76] Tagluk ME, Sezgin N, Akin M. Estimation of sleep stages by an artificial neural network employing EEG, EMG and EOG. Journal of Medical Systems. 2010;**34**:717–725. DOI 10.1007/s10916-009-9286-5

[77] Chapotot F, Becq G. Automated sleep–wake staging combining robust feature extraction, artificial neural network classification, and flexible decision rules. International Journal of Adaptive Control and Signal Processing. 2009;**1**:1–15. DOI: 10.1002/acs.1147

[78] Charbonnier S, Zoubek L, Lesecq S, Chapotot F. Self-evaluated automatic classifier as a decision-support tool for sleep/wake staging. Computers in Biology and Medicine. 2011;**41**:380–389. DOI:10.1016/j.compbiomed.2011.04.001

[79] Álvarez-Estévez D, Moret-Bonillo V. Model comparison for the detection of EEG arousals in sleep apnea patients. In: Bio-Inspired Systems: Computational and Ambient Intelligence, Volume 5517 of the series Lecture Notes in Computer Science. Berlin, Heidelberg: Springer; 2009. pp. 997–1004. DOI: 10.1007/978-3-642-02478-8_125

[80] Acharya UR, Chua EC-P, Chua KC, Min LC, Tamura T. Analysis and automatic identification of sleep stages using higher order spectra. International Journal of Neural Systems. 2010;**20:**509. DOI: 10.1142/S0129065710002589

[81] Pan S-T, Kuo C-E, Zeng J-H, Liang S-F. A transition-constrained discrete hidden Markov model for automatic sleep staging. BioMedical Engineering OnLine. 2012;**11**:52. DOI: 10.1186/1475-925X-11-52

[82] Ebrahimi F, Setarehdan S-K, Ayala-Moyeda J, Nazeran H. Automatic sleep staging using empirical mode decomposition, discrete wavelet transform, time-domain, and nonlinear dynamics features of heart rate variability signals. Computer Methods and Programs in Biomedicine. 2013;**112**:47–57. DOI: 10.1016/j.cmpb.2013.06.007

[83] Krakovská A, Mezeiová K. Automatic sleep scoring: A search for an optimal combination of measures. Artificial Intelligence in Medicine. 2011;**53:**25–33. DOI: 10.1016/j.artmed.2011.06.004

[84] Koley B, Dey D. An ensemble system for automatic sleep stage classification using single channel EEG signal. Computers in Biology and Medicine. 2012;**42:**1186–1195. DOI: 10.1016/j.compbiomed.2012.09.012

[85] Patel M, Lal SKL, Kavanagh D, Rossiter P. Applying neural network analysis on heart rate variability data to assess driver fatigue. Expert Systems with Applications. 2011;**38:**7235–7242. DOI: 10.1016/j.eswa.2010.12.028

[86] Lin C-T, Ko L-W, Chung I-F, Huang T-Y, Chen Y-C, Jung T-P, Liang S-F. Adaptive EEG-based alertness estimation system by using ICA-based fuzzy neural networks. IEEE Transactions on Circuits and Systems. 2006;**53**:2469–2476. DOI:10.1109/TCSI.2006.884408

[87] Kurt MB, Sezgin N, Akin M, Kirbas G, Bayram M. The ANN-based computing of drowsy level. Expert Systems with Applications. 2009;**36:**2534–2542. DOI: 10.1016/j.eswa.2008.01.085

[88] Garcés A, Orosco L, Laciar E. Automatic detection of drowsiness in EEG records based on multimodal analysis. Medical Engineering & Physics. 2014;**36**:244–249. DOI: 10.1016/j.medengphy.2013.07.011

[89] Dong Y, Hu Z, Uchimura K, Murayama N. Driver inattention monitoring system for intelligent vehicles: A review. IEEE Transactions on Intelligent Transportation Systems. 2011;**12**:596–614. DOI:10.1109/TITS.2010.2092770

[90] Sahayadhas A, Sundaraj K, Murugappan M. Detecting driver drowsiness based on sensors: A review. Sensors. 2012;**12**:16937–16953. DOI:10.3390/s121216937

[91] DababnehRelated L, El-GindyRelated M. Driver vigilance level detection systems: a literature survey. International Journal of Vehicle Performance. 2016;**2**:1–29. DOI: 10.1504/IJVP.2015.074120

[92] Gharibeh T, Mehra R. Obstructive sleep apnea syndrome: natural history, diagnosis and emerging treatment options. Nature and Science of Sleep 2010;**2**:233–55. DOI: 10.2147/NSS.S6844

[93] Norman RG, Rapoport DM, Ayappa I. Detection of flow limitation in obstructive sleep apnea with an artificial neural network. Physiological Measurement. 2007;**28**:1089. DOI: 10.1088/0967-3334/28/9/010

[94] Hertegonne K, Bauters F. The value of auto-adjustable CPAP devices in pressure titration and treatment of patients with obstructive sleep apnea syndrome. Sleep Medicine Reviews. 2010;**14**:115–119. DOI: 10.1016/j.smrv.2009.07.001

[95] Eklund O, Bergfalk H, Hedner JA, Knagenhjelm HP. Auto CPAP. Patent assignee: Breas Medical AB. United States Patent Number: US6889691, 2005.

[96] Waxman J, Graupe D, Carley DW. Detection and prediction of physiological events in people with sleep disordered breathing using a LAMSTAR neural network. Patent assignee: The Board of Trustees of the University of Illinois. United States Patent Number: US8775340, 2014.

[97] Hedner J, Knagenhjelm P, Tiedje M, Grote L. Multilevel ventilator. Patent assignee: Breas Medical AB. European Patent Number: EP1750581, 2014.

[98] Ayappa I, Norman RG, Whiting D, Tsai AHW, Anderson F, Donnely E, Silberstein DJ, Rapoport DM. Irregular respiration as a marker of wakefulness during titration of CPAP. Sleep. 2009;**32**:99–104.

[99] Dungan II GC, Marshall NS, Hoyos CM, Yee BJ, Grunstein RR. A randomized crossover trial of the effect of a novel method of pressure control (SensAwake) in automatic continuous positive airway pressure therapy to treat sleep disordered breathing. Journal of Clinical Sleep Medicine 2011;7:261–267. DOI: 10.5664/JCSM.1066

[100] El-Solh AA, Aldik Z, Alnabhan M, Grant B. Predicting effective continuous positive airway pressure in sleep apnea using an artificial neural network. Sleep Medicine. 2007;**8**:471–477.

[101] El-Solh AA, Akinnusi M, Patel A, Bhat A, Tenbrock R. Predicting optimal CPAP by neural network reduces titration failure: a randomized study. Sleep & Breathing. 2009;**13**:325–330. DOI: 10.1007/s11325-009-0247-5

[102] Álvarez D, Hornero R, Marcos JV, Wessel N, Penzel T, Glos M, Del Campo F. Assessment of feature selection and classification approaches to enhance information from overnight oximetry in the context of sleep apnea diagnosis. International Journal of Neural Systems. 2013;**23**:1–18. DOI: 10.1142/S0129065713500202

[103] Al-Angari HM, Sahakian AV. Automated recognition of obstructive sleep apnea syndrome using support vector machine classifier. IEEE Transactions on Information Technology in Biomedicine. 2012;**16**:463–468. DOI: 10.1109/TITB.2012.2185809

[104] Fekr AR, Janidarmian M, Radecka K, Zilic Z. A medical cloud-based platform for respiration rate measurement and hierarchical classification of breath disorders. Sensors. 2014;**14**:11204–11224. DOI: 10.3390/s140611204

[105] Lee BG, Lee BL, Chung WY. Mobile healthcare for automatic driving sleep-onset detection using wavelet-based EEG and respiration signals. Sensors. 2014;**14**:17915–17936. DOI: 10.3390/s141017915

[106] Xie B, Minn H. Real-time sleep apnea detection by classifier combination. IEEE Transactions on Information Technology in Biomedicine. 2012;**16**:469–477. DOI: 10.1109/TITB.2012.2188299

[107] Gutiérrez-Tobal GC, Álvarez D, Del Campo F, Hornero R. Utility of AdaBoost to detect sleep apnea-hypopnea syndrome from single-channel airflow. IEEE Transactions on Biomedical Engineering. 2016;**63**:636–646. DOI: 10.1109/TBME.2015.2467188

Chapter 4

Obstructive Sleep Apnea: Beyond Obesity

Rajiv Garg, Anand Srivastava and
Jagadeesha N. Halekote

Additional information is available at the end of the chapter

http://dx.doi.org/10.5772/67587

Abstract

Sleep disorders are of growing concern and are a major public health problem. The obstructive sleep apnea (OSA) is the most common among different sleep-related breathing disorders (SRBDs). Obesity is a known associated risk factor for the OSA but is not limited to them. OSA is also recognized in nonobese population. The description of OSA in non obese patients in the literature is sparse. The clinical presentation is similar as in obese but has few differences as far as pathophysiology and polysomnographic features are concerned. The severity of OSA in nonobese has less severe manifestations thus requires early recognition and different treatment strategy to prevent mismanagement of these patients.

Keywords: OSA, UARS, nonobese

1. Introduction

Sleep disorders are of growing concern and has become a major public health problem. Sleep disorders involve difficulty in breathing during sleep and are grouped under sleep-related breathing disorders (SRBDs). SRBDs are commonly classified as central sleep apnea syndrome, obstructive sleep apnea syndrome, hypoventilation/hypoxia syndrome, nonspecific/undefined sleep disorder [1]. Among SRBDs, obstructive sleep apnea (OSA) is the most common. OSA has characteristically been associated with obesity and lack of awareness and ignorance has contributed more to its increasing prevalence. OSA escaped the thought of many doctors till it was first described by Gastaut in a *Neurology journal* in 1965. Although it was first observed and mentioned in a book of Charles Dickens, an English book writer, in 1936 about a character of a person by name Joe (fat boy) in his book, *The Pickwick Papers* [2]. According to Dacal Quintas et al. [3], frequency and severity of OSA in normal weight patients was lower than overweight and obese patients. They reported frequency of 70.52 and 22% OSA in obese and normal weight patients, respectively. Normal weight group patients were mainly women, snorers, nonsmokers, nondrinkers and were significantly younger and with a smaller neck and waist circumference. The exact and recent data regarding prevalence of OSA in nonobese are not available. However, the recent studies have shown a wide scope for the evaluation of the OSA among nonobese patients globally and in India. Physicians noticed that the clinical presentations of OSA are not only limited in obese but also found in nonobese [4]. The common clinical presentation in obese and nonobese is the outcome of the basic underlying pathophysiological change that is airway narrowing or collapse during the sleep which may have different determinants that are being addressed in this chapter.

2. Pathophysiology of airway obstruction

OSA is a major public health problem affecting sizeable population. The patho physiological mechanism of OSA is not thoroughly understood and it appears to be of multifactorial origin which majorly involves interaction between anatomical (static), functional (dynamic), and systemic factors. Although these factors form the basis of OSA in nonobese and obese persons, their contribution may differ in the two groups of people.

3. Mechanism of airway obstruction during sleep

Pharynx is the only collapsible segment of the respiratory tract (except nares and small airways), and it is also the site for upper airway closure or narrowing during sleep. The patency of the pharynx is maintained by two counteracting forces, i.e. upper airway muscles (dilates and stiffens the pharynx) and negative intraluminal pressure (tends to narrow the pharynx). The imbalance between these two is the basis for OSA. Retropalatal and retroglossal areas of oropharynx are the commonly involved site in the narrowing of airways in OSA [5, 6].

The reasons for narrowing in OSA are different in nonobese and obese patients in comparison with normal individual [7]. In OSA, upper airway soft tissue enlargement may play a more important role in obese patients, whereas bony structure discrepancies may be the dominant contributing factors among nonobese patients. The various factors responsible for OSA in nonobese are mentioned below (**Figure 1**).

3.1. Anatomical (Static) factors in upper airway structure

(1) Edema: Negative pressure due to airway closure and repeated apnea may lead to edema of soft tissues particularly uvula and genioglossus [8–10].

(2) Muscle injury: Repeated fatigue of upper airway muscles in sleep apnea leads to myopathy which in turn results in remodeling of muscles [11, 12].

(3) Gender: Upper airway size and neck size are smaller in women than in men, thus the size of soft tissue structures is also smaller in women than in men. Fat deposition in men is primarily seen in upper body and trunk, whereas in women fat is deposited more commonly in lower body and extremities [13–15].

The above factors contribute to the development of OSA in both obese and nonobese. Obesity is a major risk factor for OSA, where there is decrease in pharyngeal airway size and increases airway collapsibility. Increase in neck size associated with an increase in BMI, seen in OSA patients, is a good predictor of sleep apnea. Weight gain is associated with generalized fat deposition, which contributes to the increase in the oropharyngeal muscle mass responsible for its malfunctioning and thus airway collapsibility [16–18].

3.2. Physiological (dynamic) factors in upper airway structure

The data indicate that the upper airway collapsibility during apneic events occurs at the end of expiration in addition to collapse during inspiration [19, 20]. During wakefulness, the

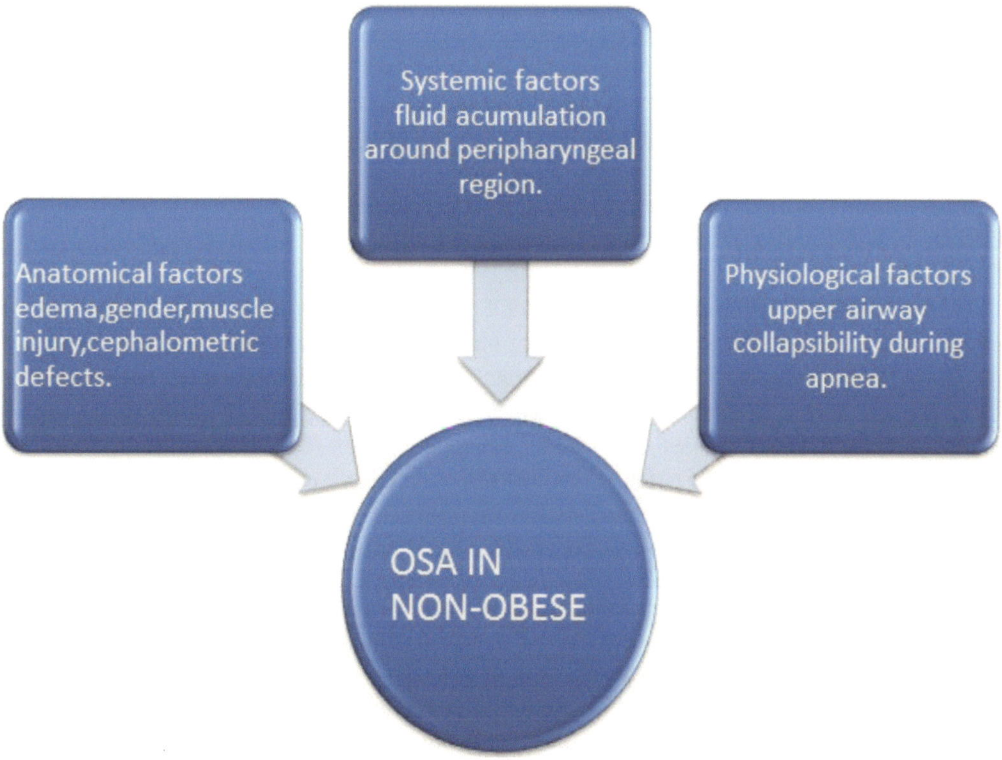

Figure 1. Factors responsible for OSA in nonobese.

balance between the upper airway dilator muscles and negative intraluminal pressure leads to a constant upper airway caliber [21, 22]. During sleep (in normal subject), it is associated with narrowing of pharyngeal luminal area due to decrease in upper airway muscle activity and a persistence of subatmospheric luminal pressure during inspiration. When the severity of this narrowing increases along with the anatomical impairment, this may lead to the development of OSA during sleep.

3.3. Systemic factors affecting upper airway structure

Accumulated fluid in the leg has a tendency to suffer overnight rostral displacement to the parapharyngeal region. Additionally, this rostral fluid displacement further interacts with the displacement of subcutaneous tissue, thus compromising the pharyngeal airway lumen. Few published articles, all in nonobese subjects, confirmed overnight increase in neck circumference resulting from shift of fluid from the legs [23–25]. This has further been proved by experimental studies using medical antishock trousers (MAST) [26, 27]. Organ failures such as heart failure [28], renal failure [29], and other disease conditions such as hypertension [30–32], stroke [33, 34], pulmonary arterial hypertension [35], and other conditions with potential for fluid retention are associated with OSA.

3.4. Other factors

Upper airway resistance syndrome (UARS) can be considered as the other factor, though the debate has been in existence since Guilleminault et al. first described UARS in 1993 [36]. The UARS has clinical presentations similar to OSA but certain differences are found in OSA and UARS. Many authors have tried to differentiate these two entities but only could reach to a very thin line of demarcation [37, 38]. The fact remains that UARS is commonly seen in nonobese, with body mass index (BMI) ≤25 kg/m^2 [39, 40]. Patients are frequently younger than patients with OSAS. UARS is more common in males but the female to male ratio seems to be highest in UARS group compared to OSA [41]. Frequent arousals due to increased respiratory effort also known as respiratory effort-related arousals (RERAs) in UARS are associated with daytime sleepiness, functional symptoms, cardiovascular, and cognitive disturbances. These RERAs are the classical features of UARS [42]. Unfortunately, many UARS patients are still under diagnosed as these patients are not subjected to polysomnographic studies as belief that patients must be obese or at least overweight with a large neck and these patients are usually labeled as fibromyalgia, chronic fatigue syndrome, or as psychiatric disorders, such as attention deficit disorder/attention deficit hyperactivity disorder (ADD/ADHD) [43].

The pathophysiology of UARS appears to be similar to OSA despite subtle differences in them. In UARS, pharyngeal reflexes are preserved compared to impaired reflexes in OSA [44]. Nocturnal polysomnography in UARS does not show apneas or hypopneas, which are the main features of obstructive sleep apnea syndrome (OSAS). Even though UARS does not have apneas/hypopneas, RERAs are associated with significant disturbances in sleep leading to impairment of daily routine of individuals. So ICSD II recommends that UARS should be considered as a part of OSA and not as a separate entity [45].

http://dx.doi.org/10.5772/67587

4. Causes for OSA in nonobese patients

Along with UARS and organ failure, causes for OSA in nonobese patients are mainly limited to several cephalometric defects compared with their BMI matched normal controls [7].

Nonobese OSA patients tend to present the following anatomical craniofacial characteristics, such as caudal hyoid, increased soft palate dimensions, and consequent anterior-posterior reductions of the airways at the soft palate level, reduction of anterior-posterior region of nasopharynx and oropharynx [7].

It has been suggested that the discrepancy in these cephalometric measurements may also depend on sex, age, and race [46–49]. OSA in Asian men has been found more frequently in the nonobese patients, despite the presence of severe illness, when compared with white male patients with OSAS [50].

Garg et al. [4] reported that nonobese subjects were more likely in habit of taking sedatives for sleeping when compared to obese counterpart, which was in concordance with other study conducted by Ghanem and Mahmood on 102 patients with OSA [51].

5. Clinical manifestations

There is no much difference between the clinical features of OSA in obese and nonobese as the pathophysiology of OSA is same in both obese and nonobese patients. Point of differentiation comes at severity of symptoms and management. Frequency and severity of OSA in nonobese is comparatively less than OSA in obese [3].

According to the study conducted by the author, the obese group had a significance with regard to lower minimal oxygen saturation (68.47 ± 13.00 vs. 80.25 ± 7.40, $P < 0.001$), higher average desaturation index (48.32 ± 13.08 vs. 30.63 ± 15.63, $P < 0.001$), and higher arousal index (28.42 ± 4.99 mm vs. 17.84 ± 5.07 mm, $P < 0.001$). Although there were a large number of obese patients than nonobese in the study (25/45 vs. 14/36) having minimum oxygen saturation <90%, the percentage of nonobese patients showing similar findings was not less (55.6 vs. 38.9, $P = 0.37$). The rest of the polysomnographic parameters were comparable [4].

6. Diagnosis

Diagnosis of OSA should be made after a comprehensive work up on the basis of history, examination, polysomnography, limited channel testing, split-night testing, and oximetry.

Since in most of these patients anatomical factors contribute to their problem, thus the emphasis should be to assess the airway thoroughly.

Airway may be assessed with the help of a number of imaging modalities such as acoustic reflexion, fluoroscopy, nasopharyngoscopy, and cephalometry (**Figures 2** and **3**; **Table 1**),

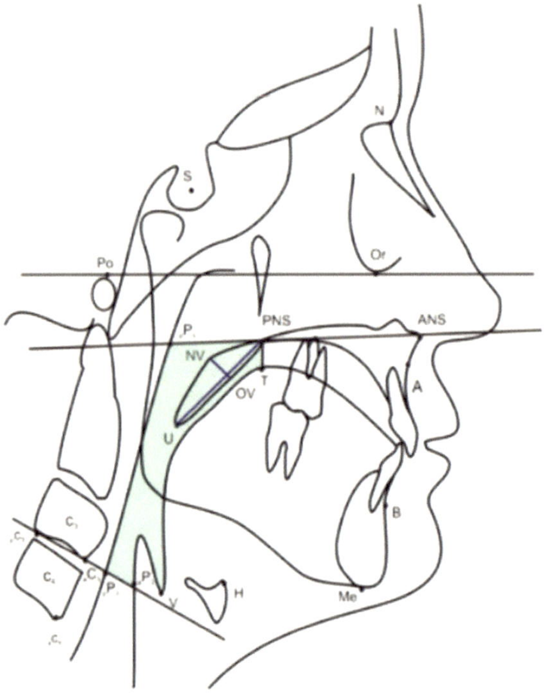

Figure 2. Cephalometric landmarks A.

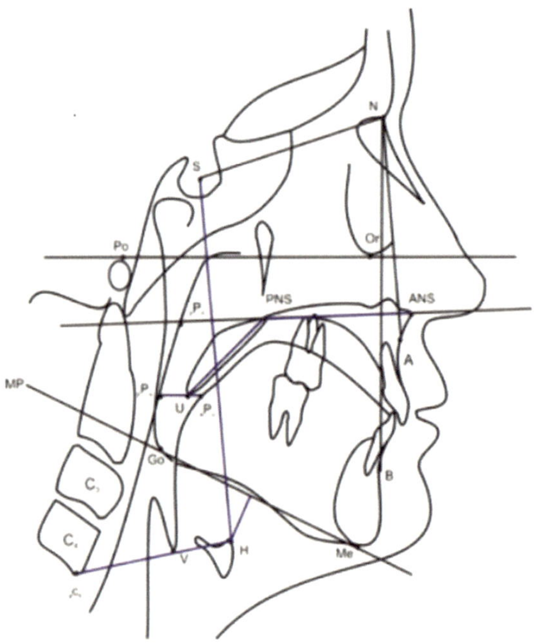

Figure 3. Cephalometric landmarks B.

S	Center of sella turcica
N	Nasion, the deepest point concavity of nasofrontal suture
ANS	Anterior nasal spine
PNS	Posterior nasal spine
Point A	The deepest point in the concavity of the anterior maxilla between the anterior nasal spine and the alveolar crest
Point B	The deepest point in the concavity of the anterior mandible between the alveolar crest and pogonion
Go	Gonion, the most posteroinferior point on angle of mandible
Me	The most inferior point on bony chin
U	The tip of uvula
OV	Intersection point between line on maximal diameter of velum in oronasal direction and oral surface of velum
NV	Intersection point between line of maximal diameter of velum in oronasal direction and nasal surface of velum
T	Intersection point between dorsal surface of tongue and line perpendicular to maxillary plane at PNS
H	The most superior and anterior point on the body of hyoid bone
${}_aC_3$	Anteroinferior point on corpus of third cervical vertebrae (C3)
${}_pC_3$	Posteroinferior point on corpus of third cervical vertebrae (C3)
${}_aC_4$	Anteroinferior point on corpus of fourth cervical vertebrae (C4)
${}_aP_u$	Intersection point between anterior pharyngeal wall and line passing through point 'U' parallel to maxillary plane
${}_pP_u$	Intersection point between posterior pharyngeal wall and line passing through point 'U' parallel to maxillary plane
${}_pP_o$	Intersection point between nasal line and posterior pharyngeal wall
${}_pP_3$	Intersection point between line connecting points, ${}_pC_3$ and ${}_aC_3$ and posterior pharyngeal wall
ANS-PNS	Maxillary plane
Go-Me	Mandibular plane (MP); line tangent to lower border of body of mandible through gnathion
H-MP	Distance between H and mandibular plane
S-H	Distance between S and H
${}_aC_4$-H	Distance between H and ${}_aC_4$
PNS-U	Soft palate length
NV-OV	Soft palate thickness
ANS-PNS-U	Soft palate (SP) angle, angle between maxillary plane and soft palate
R	Radius of curvature of nasal surface of soft palate $r = \frac{\text{(NV to OV distance)}}{2} + \frac{\text{(PNS to U distance)}^2}{8\text{(NV to OV distance)}}$
${}_aP_u - {}_pP_u$	Anteroposterior dimension of oropharynx at U
PNS-${}_pP_0$-${}_pP_3$-${}_aP_3$-L	Total pharyngeal area

Table 1. Cephalometric landmarks and reference lines used.

MR imaging, and both conventional and electron-beam CT scanning. MR imaging is probably the best imaging modality, although still not ideal [52].

7. Treatment

Possible treatment options for adult patients with OSA should be based on the severity of the sleep disorder, preference of the patient, the patient's general health, and the preference and experience of the team members. Treatment approach for OSA should be holistic and multimodality. Positive airway pressure (PAP) is universally accepted as the treatment of choice for mild, moderate, and severe OSA and thus should be offered to all patients as the first option. Side effects and adverse events are mainly minor and reversible with CPAP and BPAP therapy [53]. It may be delivered in continuous (CPAP), bilevel (BPAP), or autotitrating (APAP) modes. CPAP is indicated for the treatment of moderate-to-severe OSA [53]. Treatment of mild OSA could be optional other than PAP therapy. The American Academy of Sleep Medicine (AAOSM) has recommended the use of oral appliances (OAs) in patients with primary snoring and mild-to-moderate OSA [52]. Oral appliances are not as efficacious as CPAP. They are indicated for use in patients with mild-to-moderate OSA who prefer OAs to CPAP, or who do not respond to CPAP, are not appropriate candidates for CPAP, or who fail CPAP and are not fit candidate for surgery [54]. Oral appliances can also achieve satisfactory outcomes in UARS [55]. If surgical measures are predicted (severe obstructing anatomy that is surgically correctible) to be highly effective in treating sleep apnea, upper airway surgery (including tonsillectomy and adenoidectomy, craniofacial operations, and tracheostomy) may also supersede use of OAs. Surgical procedures may also be considered as a secondary treatment for OSA when the patient is intolerant of PAP, or PAP therapy is unable to eliminate OSA [56]. There are no widely effective pharmacotherapies for OSA. Topical nasal corticosteroids may improve the AHI in patients with OSA and concurrent rhinitis, and thus may be a useful adjunct to primary therapies for OSA. However, short-acting nasal decongestants are not recommended for treatment of OSA [56]. Oxygen supplementation has no role as a primary treatment for OSA [57]. Modafinil is recommended for the treatment as an add-on therapy of residual excessive daytime sleepiness in OSA patients who have sleepiness despite effective PAP treatment and who are lacking any other identifiable and correctable cause for their sleepiness [57]. We suggest that CPAP and Bi level is not the only modality of treatment. Any patient with systemic disorder requires treatment of primary disorder before application of these devices.

8. Conclusion

The severity of OSA in nonobese has less severe manifestation and requires different treatment strategy according to the contributory factor playing in its causation. Patients also require thorough clinical evaluation and confirmation by means of polysomnographic studies as many patients showing features of daytime sleepiness and fatigue may be erroneously managed as psychological symptoms.

The OSA in nonobese can be missed in elderly patients who have comorbidities like cardiovascular and neurological disease along with weak oropharyngeal muscles leading to easy collapsibility of airway along with obstruction. Correction of OSA in nonobese person is a multimodality approach. Assessment of upper airway anatomical variation from normalcy is a crucial step of management. Besides maintenance of sleep hygiene, patient could be subjected to many different modality of treatment as a holistic approach.

Acknowledgements

Special thanks to Dr. Deeksha Arya, Associate Professor, Department of Prosthodontics, King George's Medical University, Lucknow, for giving her valuable inputs and relevant contents.

Author details

Rajiv Garg*, Anand Srivastava and Jagadeesha N. Halekote

*Address all correspondence to: rajivkgmc@gmail.com

Department of Respiratory Medicine, King George's Medical University, Lucknow, India

References

[1] Tsara V, Amfilochiou A, Papagrigorakis MJ, et al. Guidelines for diagnosing and treating sleep related breathing disorders in adults and children. Hippokratia. 2009;13(4):247–252.

[2] Farokh EU, Zarir FU, Anirudh FK. Sleep related breathing disorders, In: *Principles of Respiratory Medicine*. Oxford, England:Oxford University Press; 2010. pp. 775–784.

[3] Dacal Quintas R, Tumbeiro Novoa M, Alves Perez MT, Santalla Martinez ML, Acuria Fernandez A, Marcos Velazquez P. Obstructive sleep apnea in normal weight patients: characteristics and comparison with overweight and obese patients. Arch Bronconeumol. 2013 Dec;49(12):5137.

[4] Garg R, Singh A, Prasad R, Saheer S, Jabeed P, Verma R. A comparative study on the clinical and polysomnographic pattern of obstructive sleep apnea among obese and non-obese subjects. Ann Thorac Med. 2012 Jan;7(1):26–30.

[5] Horner RL, Shea SA, McIvor J, Guz A. Pharyngeal size and shape during wakefulness and sleep in patients with obstructive sleep apnoea. Q J Med. 1989 Aug;72:719–735.

[6] Schwab RJ, Goldberg AN. Upper airway assessment: radiographic and other imaging techniques. Otolaryngol Clin North Am. 1998 Dec;31:931–968.

[7] Sakakibara H, Tong M, Matsushita K, Hirata M, Konishi Y, Suetsugu S. Cephalometric abnormalities in non-obese and obese patients with obstructive sleep apnoea. Eur Respir J. 1999 Feb;13(2):403–410.

[8] Ryan CF, Lowe AA, Li D, Fleetham JA. Three-dimensional upper airway computed tomography in obstructive sleep apnea. A prospective study in patients treated by uvulopalatopharyngoplasty. Am Rev Respir Dis. 1991 Aug;144:428–432.

[9] Schwab RJ. Upper airway imaging. Clin Chest Med. 1998 Mar;19:33–54.

[10] Schotland HM, Insko EK, Schwab RJ. Quantitative magnetic resonance imaging demonstrates alterations of the lingual musculature in obstructive sleep apnea. Sleep. 1999;22:605–613.

[11] Schwab, Richard J. Imaging for the snoring and sleep apnea patient. Dent Clin N Am. 2001;45:759–796.

[12] Carrera M, Barbe F, Sauleda J, Tomas M, Gomez C, Agusti AG. Patients with obstructive sleep apnea exhibit genioglossus dysfunction that is normalised after treatment with continuous positive airway pressure. Am J Respir Crit Care Med. 1999 Jun;159:1960–1966.

[13] Brooks LJ, Strohl KP. Size and mechanical properties of the pharynx in healthy men and women. Am Rev Respir Dis. 1992 Dec;146:1394–1397.

[14] Legato MJ. Gender specific aspects of obesity. Int J Fertil Womens Med. 1997 May–Jun; 42:184–197.

[15] Millman RP, Carlisle CC, McGarvey ST, Eveloff SE, Levinson PD. Body fat distribution and sleep apnea severity in women. Chest. 1995 Feb;107:362–366.

[16] Bliwise DL, Feldman DE, Bliwise NG, et al. Risk Factors for sleep disordered breathing in heterogenous geriatric populations. J Am Geriatric Soc. 1987;35:132–141.

[17] Hill JO, Sparling PB, Shields TW, Heller PA. Effects of exercise and food restriction on body composition and metabolic rate in obese women. Am J Clin Nutr. 1987 Oct;46:622–630.

[18] Wadden TA, Foster GD, Letizia KA, Mullen JL. Long term effects of dieting on resting metabolic rate in obese outpatients. JAMA. 1990 Aug;264:707–711.

[19] Schwab RJ, Gupta KB, Gefter WB, Metzger LJ, Hoffman EA, Pack AI. Upper airway and soft tissue anatomy in normal subjects and patients with sleep-disordered breathing. Significance of the lateral pharyngeal walls. Am J Respir Crit Care Med. 1995 Nov;152(5 Pt 1):1673–1689.

[20] Badr MS, Toiber F, Skatrud JB, Dempsey J. Pharyngeal narrowing/occlusion during central sleep apnea. J Appl Physiol 1995 May;78:1806–1815.

[21] Schwab RJ, Gefter WB, Pack AI, Hoffman EA. Dynamic imaging of the upper airway during respiration in normal subjects. J Appl Physiol 1993 Apr;74:1504–1514.

[22] Schwab RJ, Gefter WB, Hoffman EA, Gupta KB, Pack AI. Dynamic upper airway imaging during awake respiration in normal subjects and patients with sleep disordered breathing. Am Rev Respir Dis. 1993 Nov;148:1385–1400.

[23] Redolfi S, Yumino D, Ruttanaumpawan P, Yau B, Su MC, Lam J, Bradley TD. Relationship between overnight rostral fluid shift and Obstructive Sleep Apnea in nonobese men. Am J Respir Crit Care Med. 2009 Feb;179:241–246.

[24] Yumino D, Redolfi S, Ruttanaumpawan P, Su MC, Smith S, Newton GE, Mak S, Bradley TD. Nocturnal rostral fluid shift;a unifying concept for the pathogenesis of obstructive and central sleep apnea in men with heart failure. Circulation. 2010 Apr;121(14):1598–1605.

[25] Redolfi S, Arnulf I, Pottier M, Bradley TD, Similowski T. Effects of venous compression of the legs on overnight rostral fluid shift and obstructive sleep apnea. Respir Physiol Neurobiol. 2011 Mar;175(3):390–393.

[26] Chiu KL, Ryan CM, Shiota S, Ruttanaumpawan P, Arzt M, Haight JS, Chan CT, Floras JS, Bradley TD. Fluid shift by lower body positive pressure increases pharyngeal resistance in healthy subjects. Am J Respir Crit Care Med. 2006 Dec; 174:1378–1383.

[27] Su MC, Chiu KL, Ruttanaumpawan P, Shiota S, Yumino D, Redolfi S, Haight JS, Bradley TD. Lower body positive pressure increases upper airway collapsibility in healthy subjects. Respir Physiol Neurobiol. 2008 May;161:306–312.

[28] Sin DD, Fitzgerald F, Parker JD, Newton G, Floras JS, Bradley TD. Risk factors for central and obstructive sleep apnea in 450 men and women with congestive heart failure. Am J Respir Crit Care Med. 1991 Oct;160(4):1101–1106.

[29] Beecroft JM, Pierratos A, Hanly PJ. Clinical presentation of obstructive sleep apnea in patients with End Stage Renal Disease. J Clin Sleep Med. 2009;5(2):115–121.

[30] Haas DC, Foster GL, Nieto FJ, Redline S, Resnick HE, Robbins JA, Young T, Pickering TG. Age-dependent associations between sleep-disordered breathing and hypertension; importance of discriminating between systolic/diastolic hypertension and isolated systolic hypertension in the Sleep Heart Health Study. Circulation. 2005 Feb;111(5):614–621.

[31] Goncalves SC, Martinez D, Gus M, de Abreu-silva EO, Bertoluci C, Dutra I, Branchi T, Moreira LB, Fuchs SC, de Oliveira AC, Fuchs FD. Obstructive sleep apnea and resistant hypertension: a case control study. Chest. 2007;132(6):1858–1862.

[32] Peppard PE, Young T, Palta M, Skatrud J. Prospective study of the association between sleep-disordered breathing and hypertension. N Engl J Med. 2000 May;342(19):1378–1384.

[33] Yaggi HK, Concato J, Kernan WN, Lichtman JH, Brass LM, Mohsenin V. Obstructive sleep apnea as a risk factor for stroke and death. N Engl J Med. 2005 Nov;353(19):2034–2041.

[34] Redline S, Yenokyan G, Gottlieb DJ, Shahar E, O'Connor GT, Resnick HE, Diener -West M, Sanders MH, Wolf PA, Geraghty EM, Ali T, Lebowitz M, Punjabi NM. Obstructive sleep apnea-hypopnea and incident stroke: the sleep heart health study. Am J Respir Crit Care Med. 2010 July;182(2):269–277.

[35] Yamakawa H, Shiomi T, Sasanabe R, Hasegawa R, Ootake K, Banno K, et al. Pulmonary hypertension in patients with severe obstructive sleep apnea. Psychiatry Clin Neurosci. 2002;56(3):311–312.

[36] Palombini L, Lopes M-C, Tufik S, Christian G, Bittencourt LRA. Upper airway resistance syndrome: still not recognized and not treated. Sleep Sci. 2011;4(2):72–78.

[37] De Godoy LBM, Palombini LO, Guilleminault C, Poyares D, Tufik S, Togeiro SM. Treatment of upper airway resistance syndrome in adults: where do we stand?. Sleep Sci. 2015;8(1):42–48.

[38] De Godoy LBM, Luz GP, Palombini LO, et al. Upper airway resistance syndrome patients have worse sleep quality compared to mild obstructive sleep apnea. PLoS ONE. 2016;11(5):e0156244.

[39] Guilleminault C, Stoohs R, Clerk A, Cetel M, Maistros P. A cause of excessive daytime sleepiness . The upper airway resistance syndrome. Chest. 1993 Sep;104(3):781–7.

[40] Guilleminault C, Stoohs R, Duncan S. Snoring(I).Daytime sleepiness in regular heavy snorers. Chest . 1991 Jan;99(1):40–48.

[41] Stoohs RA, Knaack L, Blum HC, Janicki J, Hohenhorst W. Differences in clinical features of upper airway resistance syndrome, primary snoring, and obstructive sleep apnea / hypopnea syndrome. Sleep Med. 2008 Jan;9:121–128.

[42] Guilleminault C, Light D. The syndrome of the upper airway: clinical and pathophysiological relevance. Rev Respir Dis. 2005 Feb;22:27–30.

[43] Lewin DS, Di Pinto M. Sleep disorders and ADHD:shared and common phenotypes. Sleep. 2004 Mar;27(2):188–189.

[44] Pepin JL, Guillot M, Tamsier R, Levy P. The upper airway resistance syndrome. Respiration. 2012.83(6):559–566.

[45] Thorpy MJ. Classification of sleep disorders. Neurotherapeutics. 2012;9(4):687–701.

[46] Guilleminault C, Quera-Salva MA, Partinem M, Jamieson A. Women and the obstructive sleep apnea syndrome. Chest. 1988 Jan;93:104–109.

[47] Maltais F, Carrier G, Cormier Y, Series F. Cephalometric measurements in snorers, non-snorers, and patients with sleep apnea. Thorax. 1991;46:419–423.

[48] Li KK, Powell NB, Kushida C, Riley RW, Adornato B, Guilleminault C. A comparison of asian and white patients with obstructive sleep apnea syndrome. Laryngoscope. 1999 Dec;109:1937–1940.

[49] Li KK, Kushida C, Powell NB, Riley RW, Guilleminault C. Obstructive sleep apnea syndrome : a comparison between Far-East Asian and white men. Laryngoscope. 2000 Oct;110:1689–1693.

[50] Ong KC, Clerk AA. Comparison of the severityof sleep -disordered breathing in Asian and Caucasian patients seen at a sleep disorders center. Respir Med. 1998;92:843–848.

[51] Ghanem A, Mahmood S. Is obstructive sleep apnoea in non-obese patients a less serious disease than in obese patients?. Chest. 2005;128:231s-a.

[52] Padma A, Ramakrishnan N, Narayan V. Management of obstructive sleep apnea: a dental perspective. Indian J Dent Res. 2007 Oct–Dec;18(4):201–209.

[53] Kushida CA, Littner MR, Hirshkowitz M, Morgenthaler TI, Alessi CA, Bailey D, Boehlecke B, Brown TM, Coleman J Jr, Friedman L, Kapen S, Kapur VK, Kramer M, Lee-Chiong T, Owens J, Pancer JP, Swick TJ, Wise MS. Practice parameters for the use of continuous and bilevel positive airway pressure devices to treat adult patients with sleep related breathing disorders. Sleep. 2006 Mar;29:375–380.

[54] Ramar K, Dort LC, Katz SG, Lettieri CJ, Harrod CG, Thomas SM, Chervin RD. Clinical practice guideline for the treatment of Obstructive Sleep Apnea and Snoring with Oral Appliance Therapy: an update for 2015. J Clin Sleep Med. 2015 July;11(7):773–827.

[55] Yoshida K. Oral device therapy for the upper airway resistance syndrome patient. J Prosthet Dent. 2002.87(4):427–430.

[56] Kushida CA, Morgenthaler TI, Littner MR, Alessi CA, Bailey D, Coleman J Jr, Friedman L, Hirschkowitz M, Kapen S, Kramer M, Lee-chiong T, Owens J, Pancer JP. American academy of sleep. Practise parameters for the treatment of snoring and obstructive sleep apnea with oral appliances:an update for 2005. Sleep. 2006;29:240–243.

[57] Morgenthaler T, Kapen S, Lee-Chiong T, Alessi C, Boehlecke B, Brown T, Coleman J, Friedman L, Kapur V, Owens J, Pancer J, Swick T. Practice parameters for the medical therapy of obstructive sleep apnea. Sleep. 2006 Aug;29:1031–1035.

Chapter 5

Management of Obstructive Sleep Apnea by Maxillomandibular Advancement Surgery

Gurkan Rasit Bayar and Tamer Zerener

Additional information is available at the end of the chapter

http://dx.doi.org/10.5772/65437

Abstract

Obstructive sleep apnea (OSA) is a common disorder characterized by recurrent episodes of partial or complete collapsibility of upper airway during sleep. The use of nocturnal positive airway pressure that pneumatically stents open the upper airway has been considered the first-line treatment of OSA. However, in the last two decades, maxillomandibular advancement (MMA) has been widely suggested as the most effective craniofacial surgical technique for the treatment of OSA in adults. It has been shown that the pharyngeal and hypopharyngeal airway could be enlarged with MMA surgery by physically expanding the facial skeletal framework. Tissue tension could be increased by forward movement of the maxillomandibular complex. Thus, collapsibility of the velopharyngeal and suprahyoid musculature could be decreased, and lateral pharyngeal wall collapse could be improved. Recent systematic reviews and meta-analyses showed that most of the subjects reported satisfaction after MMA with improvements in quality of life (QOL) measures and most of OSA symptomatology. According to the recent updates, MMA appears to be the most successful surgical option for the treatment of OSA, and it could be an excellent alternative procedure for nonresponders, or deniers of ventilation therapy.

Keywords: obstructive sleep apnea, maxillomandibular, advancement, surgery, orthognathic surgery

1. Introduction

Obstructive sleep apnea (OSA) is a common disorder characterized by recurrent episodes of partial or complete collapsibility of upper airway during sleep. Disturbed sleep pattern and less restorative sleep owing to the recurrent hypoxia events and sleep fragmentation can lead to the symptoms of excessive daytime sleepiness, fatigue, and neurocognitive deficits. The increased risk of accidents, cardiovascular and cerebrovascular morbidity and mortality such as myocardial infarction and stroke are life-threatening sequelae. Additionally, patients may have depression, physical and intellectual impairment, erectile dysfunction, and headache [1–10]. The mortality rate for severe OSA was reported as approximately 30% at 15 years, if it is left untreated [3].

Several treatment options have been recommended to OSA patients. The use of nocturnal positive airway pressure (either continuous [CPAP] or bilevel) that pneumatically stents open the upper airway has been suggested as the reference standard treatment for the management of OSA [2–5]. However, it was reported that more than 50% of patients showed poor adherence rates, within the first few months after initiation [2, 3]. Therefore, patients' compliance problem to CPAP leads them seek surgical treatment. Surgery has been shown to be another valid option for patients who are intolerant to positive pressure therapy. The posterior airspace of OSA patients, who is intolerant to CPAP, could be successfully increased by some soft tissue surgical procedures available. Despite that, the reported surgical success rate for these procedures is approximately 40–60% [3].

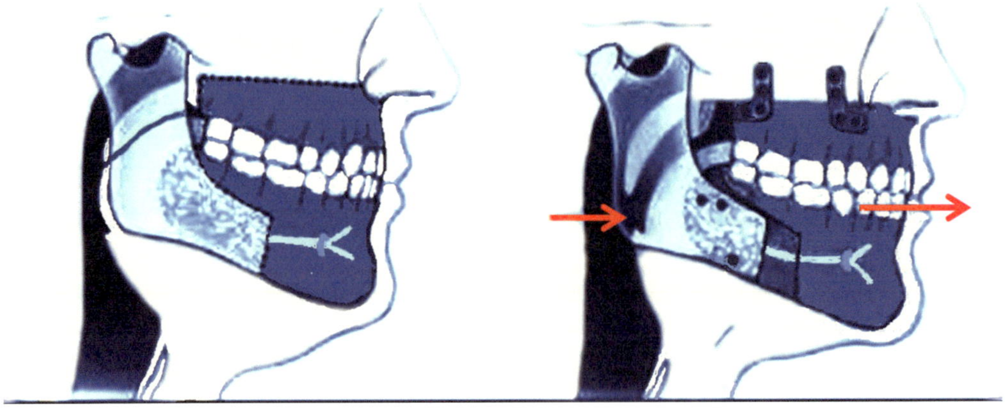

Figure 1. An illustration showing maxillomandibular advancement (MMA) surgery. Arrows show the upper and lower jaws move forward surgically and enlargement of the airway.

Another surgical treatment option for treating the patients with OSA is maxillomandibular advancement (MMA) surgery. It was suggested that MMA is currently the most effective craniofacial surgical technique for the treatment of OSA in adults [2, 7, 11]. By expanding the skeletal framework, MMA enlarges the pharyngeal space and enhances the tension of the soft tissues, reducing the collapsibility and obstruction of the pharynx (**Figure 1**) [3, 7]. This procedure is routinely performed to correct dysgnathia [7]. In the previous studies, the surgical technique and pre- and postoperative care in the treatment of OSA have been extensively described [12, 13].

In this chapter, we firstly present some basic information about MMA surgery, and then, we review the published data concerning the recent updates related to the evaluations of effectiveness of MMA surgery performed for the treatment of OSA syndrome.

2. Preoperative examination

2.1. General workup

An exact medical and sleep history should be taken regardless of patients' age. Epworth Sleepiness Scale can be used for adults [14], but it is not excellent and does not every time establish a connection with OSA violence. Head, neck, and nasopharynx examination are recommended with a lateral cephalometric head film and fiberoptic nasopharyngoscopy. Also, nasal airway obstruction, lateral pharyngeal walls, the palatal region, tonsils, malocclusions and skeletal abnormalities, tongue and tongue base should be examined. Especially, polysomnography (PSG) is very important for a diagnosis or treatment plan [15].

2.2. Polysomnography

Preoperative and postoperative polysomnography is very sensitive method which is to evaluate of surgery success rate. On the other hand, this method also indicates the success rate of the surgeon. Some of the parameters such as; age, body mass index (BMI), total sleep time, sleep stages, apnea index, hypopnea index, awake SaO2, lowest SaO2, heart rate fluctuations, and periodic leg movements should be evaluated [15, 16]. These results are expressed as the respiratory disturbance index (RDI) or the apnea-hypopnea index (AHI). An AHI of 5 or less is evaluated normal for an adult [15].

2.3. Cephalometric head film

Cephalometric head films are used in orthodontics, which evaluates soft tissue and bony anatomy. Cephalometric radiographs can also be used to understand the hard tissue and soft tissue growth rate. For this purpose, specific points, planes, and angles on the head such as sella-nasion subspinale angle (SNA), sella-nasion-supramentale angle (SNB), distance from the superior nasal spine to the tip of the soft palate (PNS-P), posterior airway space (PAS), and distance from the mandibular plane to the hyoid bone (MP-H) are used [15, 17].

2.4. Fiberoptic examination

Nasopharyngolaryngoscopy is used to determine the obstruction at the nose, retropalatal, and tongue base area. It is also used to identify upper airway obstruction causes such as tumors, cysts, and laryngeal pathology [12].

2.5. Preoperative management

A detailed history should be taken from the patient and should be determined whether there is a systemic disease. Patients who undergo bimaxillary advancement have increased risks of medical, surgical, and regarding anesthesia. For that reason, these patients regardless of age should have an exact check-up. It should be explained to the patients what they will need to do on the day before surgery. In addition, arch bars should be applied to both jaws [15].

3. Surgical stage

3.1. LeFort 1 osteotomies

Firstly, a nasal intubation is requested from the anesthetist for the MMA surgery. Following a nasotracheal intubation, hypotensive tension could be wanted from anesthetist, in order to reduce bleeding of the patient. After that, local anesthesia could be also made to reduce bleeding and gain an additional anesthesia. Surgical operation is started by a maxillary gingivobuccal incision, which is made from the first molar on one side to the first molar on the opposite side. In order to expose the anterior face of the maxilla from the piriform rims anteriorly and back to the pterygoid processes, subperiosteal dissection is performed. For the avoidance of infraorbital nerve damage, mucosa retractor has to be used safely around infraorbital nerve area. After the piriform aperture is detected, the dissection is carried out medially to the nasal spine. Then, a round bur or saw is used to make horizontal osteotomies from the nasal apertures to the pterygomaxillary fissures bilaterally. Tooth apexes should be watched out during horizontal osteotomies. After that, osteotome is used to separate the nasal septum from the maxillary crest. Finally, using a curved osteotome the pterygoid plates are separated from the tuberosities of the maxilla. While doing this osteotome, one finger should be placed in the oropharynx at the level of the hamulus, in order to obtain a bimanual tactile feedback. To refrain injuring of the pterygoid plexus, osteotome must be put correct position on the pterygoid plate's areas. Then, downfracture is made and maxilla mobilized. The descending palatine arteries are checked out and preserved. If necessary, medial wall of the maxilla and other anatomical bone structures are shaved and removed according to the maxillary advancement and impaction planned. Adequate mobility must be acquired to advance the jaw passively into the requested position, which in many patients with OSA is around 10 mm. Rigid fixation of the maxilla is done with four titanium L-shaped four-holes miniplates (two per side) using 2.0 × 5 mm mono-cortical screws. An intermediate guide splint is frequently useful here to adjust the maxillary position and prevent midline disagreements and vertical faults of the jaw [17].

3.2. Bilateral sagittal split osteotomies

After local anesthesia, an incision is made throughout the external oblique ridge from midramus height to the mandibular first molar. Subperiosteal flap is raised to expose the lateral border of the mandible and anterior aspect of the ramus. Muscle on the medial part of the ramus is stripped high enough on the coronoid process to access to the mandibular foramen and lingual process. The Hunsack modification of the Obwegeser and DalPont bilateral split sagittal osteotomy technique is applied [17]. Using lingula recractor, 4–5 mm horizontal osteotomy is made with a saw or burr until to just behind and above of the lingula. Osteotomy is made half way through the thickness of the bone, and parallel to the occlusal plane. Continuing osteotomy is made inferiorly with a sagittal saw blade along the anterior border of the ascending ramus till to the level of the first molar (remaining 5 mm lateral to the teeth). Then, the vertical osteotomy is performed on the buccal cortex, in a vertical direction near to the first molar, and is extended down to the inferior border. At the inferior border, the osteotomy must be completed to include both inner and outer cortices. The osteotomy should be extended superiorly at least 5 mm or more at the inner cortice of the mandible; otherwise, the bad split might be occurred. Osteotomes are used to track the osteotomy site throughout the entire length of the cuts, after that spreader is used to complete the splits on both sides of the mandible. Then, the inferior alveolar nerve must be detected, and if it is in the lateral segment, inferior alveolar nerve must be entrenched into the medial segment of the mandible. Surgical sites are abundantly irrigated and the throat pack is removed. The same surgical protocols applied for the opposite side. The correct position of the jaw is achieved by using the final splint. Maxillomandibular fixation is made by intermaxillary wires. Medial and lateral fragments of the mandible are fixed with three bi-cortical screws through intraoral and percutaneous approaches. Titanium plate/plates could be also placed and secured with mono-cortical screws. After that, intermaxillary fixation is solved by cutting the wires and the final splint is removed from the mouth. The mandibular movements and occlusion is checked. Bleeding is controlled, and then, soft tissues are sutured with 3-0 silk or chromic sutures. Finally, to avoid relapse, six or eight ounce elastic bands are placed and a head dressing is applied [17].

4. Postoperative evaluations

Patients with OSA who underwent MMA surgery stay mostly overnight in the intensive care unit (ICU). The use of CPAP could be useful, particularly when the patients are sleeping, to maintain the opening of airway, control of edema, and lessen the use of narcotics [15, 17]. Antibiotics, analgesics, steroids, and mouth rinse are prescribed. Higher lying position (around 30–45°) is set, and intravenous fluids are given. Application of ice is recommended in the first 48 h. Rigid fixation is not recommended because of the possibility of vomiting and airway obstruction. Advancement of the patients' diet consist of intravenous fluids for the first 24 h, then a full liquid diet is launched for a week, and followed by a no chew diet for 5–6 weeks. Discharge of the patient from the hospital is evaluated according to the absence of some parameters such as; fewer, pain, oral intake, surgeon, and patient's opinions. Generally, hospitalization time is 2–3 days for an adult OSA patient, who is underwent a bimaxillary procedure. Using of CPAP could be advised to the patients while sleeping until the follow-up plysomnography. The follow-up plysomnography is generally performed between the 4th and 6th months postoperatively [17]. If everything goes well, periodic controls are made at every 6 months for the first year, and then yearly.

5. Recent updates in management of obstructive sleep apnea by maxillomandibular advancement surgery

To date, MMA has been suggested as the most effective surgical treatment option available for OSA by sufficient number of published data [1–8]. Also, it was reported that MMA could possibly be the definitive primary single-stage option for the treatment of OSA in selected patients [2].

In 2010, Holty and Guilleminault at the end of their meta-analysis including 22 studies of 627 adult OSA subjects treated by MMA reported four key findings [3]. Firstly, they suggested that MMA is highly effective at treating OSA. They found that the mean AHI decreased from 63.9/h to 9.5/h with a pooled surgical success rate of 86.0%. Moreover, they specified that long-term surgical success was maintained at a mean follow-up of 44 months. Secondly, it was stated that the surgical success with univariate or multivariate analysis would not be predicted by the degree of mandibular advancement. Thirdly, it was concluded that MMA was generally safe procedure for treating OSA with a reported major surgical complication rate of 1.0% and minor complication rate of 3.1% and no reported deaths. Malocclusion (up to 44%) and persistent facial paresthesias (14.2% at one year) were also reported. Fourthly, satisfaction with the surgical outcome with few noting aesthetic complaints were reported by the most of subjects. After MMA, improvements in quality of life measures, OSA symptomatology (i.e., excessive daytime sleepiness), and blood pressure control were statistically significant [3].

Li [2] reported more than 600 MMAs for the treatment of OSA, with a success rate of 89% till 2011. This report was consistent with the published data and the results from the meta-analysis by Holty and Guilleminault [3]. Li [2] asserted that younger age and a lower BMI would be predictors for greater surgical success, as long as sufficient advancement could be performed. On the other hand, negative predictors were reported as older age (upper than 60 years), greater BMI (upper than 33 kg/m^2), and limited advancement. Probable poor candidates for surgery were specified as obese patients with white fat accumulation and abnormal adipocyte activity, or those with a long disease duration with a greater risk of permanent neurologic deficits in the pharyngeal airway. However, it was also reported that patients with negative predictors could experience significant improvement. Thus, a dramatic resolution on the symptoms could be obtained in the most of patients with some residual OSA on polysomnography. In spite of that, a few patients with minimal improvement despite a very successful operation with 15-mm advancement were reported [2].

Thus, though good outcomes could be obtained, successful outcomes might not be achieved in all patients. Therefore, the complexity of OSA should be accepted. As a result, it must be recognized that a 100% success rate should not be claimed by any surgeon. Moreover, the major concern of MMA surgery should be the associated risks, as with any surgical intervention. Conclusively, followings are essential to achieve an ideal and successful outcome; performing of proper surgical methods with adequate advancement and fixation techniques, management of the soft tissue changes without compromising the esthetic results, and precautionary in airway management [2].

In order to achieve greater advancement with minimal adverse esthetic effects, certain reserachers have also tried to modify surgical techniques. For example, Bruno-Carlo et al. [18] described monocortical genioplasty, and segmentectomy after premolar extraction in both jaws was performed by Goh et al. [19].

In another systematic review of 39 studies conducted by Pirklbauer et al. [7], maxillomandibular advancement was reported as the most successful surgical therapy. Also, the postoperative polysomnography results were comparable to those under ventilation therapy. According to their results, recently MMA was preferred as a primary intervention by more investigators than had been done in the past. Thus, they concluded that OSAS patients with skeletal deficiency could benefit from MMA as a primary surgical intervention and do not need be subjected to less successful surgical procedures [7].

Because sleep endoscopy during spontaneous sleep does not seem applicable in routine clinical practice, airway endoscopy with pharmacologic sedation, or druginduced sleep endoscopy (DISE) was described [20]. Dynamic evaluation of the airway during drug-induced sleep using endoscopy has increased in popularity and also proved to be an important tool in predicting the outcome of upper airway surgery for patients with OSA [21, 22]. It is still inconclusive whether drug-induced sleep could be generalized to natural sleep. On the other hand, it is obvious that DISE can allow to observe the dynamic airway activity in real time.

It was reported that MMA expands the skeletal frame attached with the pharyngeal structures and tongue. Thus, it results in an increased upper airway space by reducing airway collapsibility during negative-pressure inspiration [3, 23, 24].

Before, the intrapharyngeal changes after MMA had only been studied using static imaging and endoscopy of subjects who were awake. In 2015, Liu et al. [23] aimed to characterize the patterns of dynamic airway collapse during sleep endoscopy for subjects before and after MMA. At the end of their study, their results showed that the tension in the lateral pharyngeal wall increased significantly after MMA and the change correlated highly with surgical success. They reported that the tension in the lateral pharyngeal wall would contribute more to success than did the changes at the palate or tongue base. As a result, they concluded that the subjects without a history of intrapharyngeal soft tissue surgery (palatal or tongue) had greater improvement in the AHI [23].

In 2016, Faria et al. [25] also compared the dynamic differences occurring in the pharynx during sleep after MMA surgery for the treatment of patients with OSA. This was a prospective, cross-sectional study. Twenty patients (fifteen men and five women) were submitted to magnetic resonance (MR) during propofol-induced sleep before and six months after surgery. Then, their variability before and after MMA were compared. During induced sleep after MMA, 66% mean linear anteroposterior increase of the pharynx was reported in the retrolingual region. It was specified that the coefficient of variation of the linear measurements was reduced from 117.5 to 51 % after surgery. At the end of the study, it was concluded that MMA promoted an important increase in the pharynx during induced sleep. Also, the diameter of the organ was with a lower variation during the respiratory movements. Thus, there was greater airway stability and a consequent maintenance of the pharyngeal lumen that reduces or even prevents pharyngeal collapse [25].

In another meta-analysis conducted in 2015, comparison of the patients with OSA who undergo MMA with counterclockwise (CCW) rotation and those who undergo MMA without CCW rotation was investigated by Knudsen et al. [26]. Consequently, they reported that CCW-MMA or MMA in patients with OSA resulted in a statistically meaningful decrease in postoperative AHI and a statistically meaningful increase in postoperative lowest oxygen saturation (LSAT) [26].

Another important issue is that the comprehensive examination of the long-term effectiveness and safety of MMA as an alternative therapy to CPAP. In 2015, Boyd et al. [5] conducted a study to determine if MMA is a clinically effective and safe long-term treatment for OSA patients by measuring the changes in the AHI, blood pressure, sleepiness, and QOL. Their results showed that MMA produces substantial and sustained reductions in the diastolic blood pressure, and subjective sleepiness, AHI with accompanying improvements in QOL. It was important that MMA had a good risk-benefit ratio, as these successful outcomes had been achieved in the context of minimal long-term treatment-related adverse outcomes. They concluded that the results of their study provided compelling evidence to suggest that MMA should be the alternative treatment of choice for patients with severe OSA who cannot fully adhere to CPAP [5].

Beside many studies regarding long-term effectiveness and safety of MMA surgery for the management of obstructive sleep apnea (OSA), the subjective effect of this treatment modality was also investigated by Butterfield et al. [4] in 2016. In this study, quantification of the subjective change in QOL in patients who had undergone MMA for the management of OSA; assessment of the effect of the treatment-related side effects of MMA on patient QOL; and evaluation the relationship between objective changes in OSA severity with the subjective changes in QOL were studied. Their study showed that although some patients might experience few MMA-related postoperative side effects during recovery, MMA for OSA significantly improved patient's subjective overall QOL [4].

In addition to many studies in the literature showing MMA as a safe treatment modality, there is another study dealing with detailed comparison of outcomes in OSA and dentofacial deformity (DFD) patients undergoing the same procedures. Passeri et al. [11] compared morbidity and mortality rates in OSA versus DFD patients undergoing equivalent maxillofacial surgical procedures. Their study indicated that even though the patients in the OSA group were older, had more comorbidities, and ultimately had a greater number of early, late, minor, and major complications than those in the DFD group, MMA seemed to be a safe procedure [11].

As well as many adult OSA patients, Ahn et al. [27] reported that a 11.1 years old female patient with refractory OSA (AHI score of 8.2, and RDI score of 11.6) and serious medical history (pneumonia, asthma attacks, hyperventilation-related dyspnea or tachypnea, psychosocial problems, etc.) could be treated by modified MMA surgery, accompanied by upper and lower anterior segmental osteotomies (ASOs). As a conclusion, they proposed that modified MMA surgery, combined with ASOs, could be a successful treatment alternative for a preadolescent patient with refractory OSA. They specified that postoperative improvement occurred in the affected functions and esthetics, and the improvements were stable throughout the growth period of their patient [27].

6. Conclusions

In our opinion, the recent evidences in the published data support the recommendation of MMA to treat patients with severe OSA who cannot fully adhere to CPAP.

According to the recent updates, MMA appears to be the most successful surgical option for the treatment of OSA, and it could be an excellent alternative procedure for non-responders, or deniers of ventilation therapy. However, more randomized controlled trials on larger sample sizes, and long-term investigations are needed to attain this recommendation.

Author details

Gurkan Rasit Bayar* and Tamer Zerener

*Address all correspondence to: gurkanbayar@yahoo.com

Department of Oral and Maxillofacial Surgery, Gulhane Military Medical Academy, Ankara, Turkey

References

[1] Sencimen M, Bayar GR, Akcam T, Altug HA, Altug H, Gulses A, Ozkan A: Management of obstructive sleep apnea by maxillomandibular advancement surgery in an edentulous patient. J Craniofac Surg. 2012; 23(6): e582-e584. DOI: 10.1097/SCS.0b013e3182 6befe0.

[2] Li KK: Maxillomandibular advancement for obstructive sleep apnea. J Oral Maxillofac Surg. 2011; 69: 687–694. DOI: 10.1016/j.joms.2010.09.014.

[3] Holty JEC, Guilleminault C: Maxillomandibular advancement for the treatment of obstructive sleep apnea: a systematic review and meta-analysis. Sleep Med Rev. 2010; 14: 287–297. DOI: 10.1016/j.smrv.2009.

[4] Butterfield KJ, Marks PL, McLean L, Newton J: Quality of life assessment after maxillomandibular advancement surgery for obstructive sleep apnea. J Oral Maxillofac Surg. 2016; 74(6):1228–1237. DOI:10.1016/j.joms.2016.01.043.

[5] Boyd SB, Walters AS, Waite P, Harding SM, Song Y: Long-term effectiveness and safety of maxillomandibular advancement for treatment of obstructive sleep apnea. J Clin Sleep Med. 2015; 11(7): 699–708. DOI: 10.5664/jcsm.4838.

[6] Zaghi S, Holty JEC, Certal V, Adullatif J, Guilleminault C, Powel NB, Riley RW, Camacho M: Maxillomandibular advancement for treatment of obstructive sleep apnea: a meta-analysis. JAMA Otolaryngol Head Neck Surg. 2016; 142(1): 58–66. DOI: 10.1001/jamaoto.2015.2678.

[7] Pirklbauer K, Russmueller G, Stiebellehner L, Nell C, Sinko K, Millesi G, Klug C: Maxillomandibular advancement for treatment of obstructive sleep apnea syndrome: a systematic review. J Oral Maxillofac Surg. 2011; 69: e165–e176. DOI: 10.1016/j.joms.2011.01.038.

[8] Benjamin JA, Lewis KE: Sleep-disordered breathing and cardiovascular disease. Postgrad Med. 2008; 84: 15–22. DOI: 10.1136/pgmj.2007.062836.

[9] George CF: Sleep apnea, alertness, and motor vehicle crashes. Am J Respir Crit Care Med. 2007; 176:954–956. DOI: 10.1164/rccm.200605-629PP.

[10] Yaggi HK, Concato J, Kernan WN, Lichtman JH, Brass LM, Mohsenin V. Obstructive sleep apnea as a risk factor for stroke and death. N Engl J Med. 2005; 353: 2034–2041. DOI: 10.1056/NEJMoa043104

[11] Passeri LA, Choi JG, Kaban LB, Lahey ET 3rd: Morbidity and mortality rates after maxillomandibular advancement for treatment of obstructive sleep apnea. J Oral Maxillofac Surg. 2016; Apr. 21 [Epublished ahead of print]. DOI: 10.1016/j.joms.2016.04.005.

[12] Schendel SA, Powell NB: Surgical orthognathic management of sleep apnea. J Craniofac Surg. 2007; 18: 902–911. DOI: 10.1097/scs.0b013e31806843b5.

[13] George LT, Barber HD, Smith BM: Maxillomandibular advancement surgery: an alternative treatment option for obstructive sleep apnea. Atlas Oral Maxillofac Surg Clin North Am. 2007; 15: 163–177. DOI: 10.1016/j.cxom.2007.05.006.

[14] Johns M: A new method for measuring daytime sleepiness: the Epworth sleepiness scale. Sleep. 1991; 14:540–545.

[15] Powell NB, Riley RW, Guilleminalut C: Surgical management of sleep-disordered breathing. In: Kryger MH, Roth T, Dement WC, editors. Principles and Practices of Sleep Medicine, 5th ed. Philadelphia: Elsevier Saunders; 2005. p. 1081–1097. DOI: 10.1002/ppul.1950080117.

[16] Young T, Palta M, Dempsey J, Skatrud J, Weber S, Badr S: The occurrence of sleep disordered breathing among middle-aged adults. N Engl J Med. 1993; 328: 1230–1235.

[17] Camacho M, Liu SY, Certal V, Capasso R, Powell NB, Riley RW: Large maxillomandibular advancements for obstructive sleep apnea: an operative technique evolved

over 30 years. J Craniomaxillofac Surg. 2015; 43(7): 1113–1118. DOI: 10.1016/j.jcms.2015.05.015.

[18] Bruno-Carlo B, Mauro P, Silvia B, Enrico S: Modified genioplasty and bimaxillary advancement for treating obstructive sleep apnea syndrome. J Oral Maxillofac Surg. 2008; 66: 1971–1974. DOI: 10.1016/j.joms.2008.01.051.

[19] Goh YH, Lim KA: Modified maxillomandibular advancement for the treatment of obstructive sleep apnea: a preliminary report. Laryngoscope. 2003; 113: 1577–1582. DOI: 10.1097/00005537-200309000-00031.

[20] Croft CB, Pringle M: Sleep nasendoscopy: a technique of assessment in snoring and obstructive sleep apnoea. Clin Otolaryngol Allied Sci. 1991; 16: 504–509.

[21] Ravesloot MJ, de Vries N: One hundred consecutive patients undergoing drug-induced sleep endoscopy: Results and evaluation. Laryngoscope. 2011; 121: 2710–2716. DOI: 10.1002/lary.22369.

[22] Safiruddin F, Koutsourelakis I, de Vries N: Analysis of the influence of head rotation during drug-induced sleep endoscopy in obstructive sleep apnea. Laryngoscope. 2014; 124: 2195–2199. DOI: 10.1002/lary.24598.

[23] Liu SY, Huon LK, Powell NB, Riley R, Cho HG, Torre C, Capasso R: Lateral pharyngeal wall tension after maxillomandibular advancement for obstructive sleep apnea is a marker for surgical success: observations from drug-induced sleep endoscopy. J Oral Maxillofac Surg. 2015; 73(8): 1575–1582. DOI: 10.1016/j.joms.2015.01.028.

[24] Prinsell JR: Primary and secondary telegnathic maxillomandibular advancement, with or without adjunctive procedures, for obstructive sleep apnea in adults: a literature review and treatment recommendations. J Oral Maxillofac Surg. 2012; 70: 1659–1677. DOI: 10.1016/j.joms.2011.03.064.

[25] Faria AC, Garcia LV, Santos AC, Eckeli AL, Garcia DM, Mello-Filho FV: Dynamic comparison of pharyngeal stability during sleep in patients with obstructive sleep apnea syndrome treated with maxillomandibular advancement. Sleep Breath. 2016; May 26 [Epublished ahead of print]. DOI: 10.1007/s11325-016-1362-8.

[26] Knudsen TB, Laulund AS, Ingerslev J, Homøe P, Pinholt EM: Improved apnea-hypopnea index and lowest oxygen saturation after maxillomandibular advancement with or without counterclockwise rotation in patients with obstructive sleep apnea: a meta-analysis. J Oral Maxillofac Surg. 2015; 73(4): 719–726. DOI: 10.1016/j.joms.2014.08.006.

[27] Ahn HW, Lee BS, Kim SW, Kim SJ: Stability of modified maxillomandibular advancement surgery in a patient with preadolescent refractory obstructive sleep apnea. J Oral Maxillofac Surg. 2015; 73(9): 1827–1841. DOI: 10.1016/j.joms.2015.02.028.

Chapter 6

Head Posture and Upper Cervical Spine Morphology in Patients with Obstructive Sleep Apnea

Liselotte Sonnesen

Additional information is available at the end of the chapter

http://dx.doi.org/10.5772/65436

Abstract

The main aim of this chapter is to describe the role of upper cervical spine morphology and head and neck posture in the etiology, diagnosis, and treatment in patients with obstructive sleep apnea (OSA). Previously it has been documented that the posture of the head and neck was related to the morphology of the facial profile, dysfunction of the jaws, and obstruction of the upper airway. It has been shown that head posture in relation to the upper cervical spine was extended in OSA patients. New findings have been added concerning the occurrence and pattern of deviations of the upper cervical spine morphology in OSA. Furthermore, associations between upper cervical spine morphology and the morphology of the facial profile, including the cranial base in OSA patients have been reported. In addition, the occurrence of upper cervical spine morphological deviations in OSA patients seems to affect the outcome of the treatment with a mandibular advancement devise (MAD). Accordingly, it is suggested that upper cervical spine morphology and posture of the head and neck are important factors in the etiology, diagnosis, and treatment considerations in OSA patients.

Keywords: head posture, cervical spine morphology, sleep apnea

1. Introduction

Obstructive sleep apnea (OSA) is by far the most common sleep-related breathing disorder, affecting 2–4% of the adult population, particularly males aged 60 years and older where the prevalence is 30–60% [1, 2]. OSA is defined as cessation of airflow with persistent respiratory effort, due to repeated anatomical obstruction or partial collapse of the oropharyngeal region, involving the soft palate, dorsum of the tongue, and the posterior pharyngeal wall [1, 3]. The majority of the patients have symptoms such as loud snoring and excessive daytime sleepiness [4, 5]. Nightly choking or gasping, morning headache, memory loss, decreased concentration, increased irritability, and nocturia are also reported [4, 6]. Thus, OSA has consequences for the quality of life, working ability, and traffic safety as well as comorbidities as hypertension [4–7]. OSA is multifactorial with age, gender, and body mass index (BMI) as predisposing factors [1, 3]. The authors agree that there are craniofacial morphological and postural characteristics in OSA patients such as reduced posterior airway space, abnormally long soft palate, low position of the hyoid bone, and an extended head posture [8, 9]. The primary treatments of OSA are based on physical effects and consist of continuous positive airway pressure (CPAP), mandibular advancement device (MAD), and upper airway surgery [6, 7].

This chapter focuses on the role of head posture and the morphology of the upper cervical spine in the etiology, diagnosis, and treatment in patients with OSA.

2. Head posture in relation to OSA

Associations between head posture and pharyngeal airway dimensions have been documented on lateral cephalograms [9–12]. It was found that an extension of the head in relation to the upper cervical spine resulted in an increase of the anterior-posterior dimension of the pharynx. Furthermore, studies have shown the influence of airway obstruction on head posture [9, 13, 14] where airway obstruction resulted in an extension of the head in relation to the upper cervical spine. Due to the head posture's close associations with the pharyngeal airway, it seems relevant to focus on the relationship between the head posture and OSA.

2.1. Definition of head posture

Natural head position is a standardized and reproducible position of the head in an upright position determined by the subjects' own postural control system [14–16]. Accordingly, the posture of the head and neck can be defined in two ways: with or without external reference. The "self-balance position" is without external reference (the subjects' proprioceptive system) and the "mirror position", with external reference (the subjects' proprioceptive and visual system) [13, 14]. In this chapter, the head posture refers to the OSA patients' "self-balance position" or the "mirror position" evaluated on lateral cephalograms and defined as the following angels [17–19] (**Figure 1**).

1. Posture of the head related to an environmentally determined vertical or horizontal line, that is, the cranio-vertical angles (NSL/VER, NL/VER).

2. Posture of the head related to a line representing the upper spine, that is, the cranio-cervical angles (NSL/OPT, NL/OPT, NSL/CVT, NL/CVT).

3. The upper spine inclination expressed in relation to the environmentally determined true horizontal, that is, the cervico-horizontal angles (OPT/HOR, CVT/HOR).

http://dx.doi.org/10.5772/65436

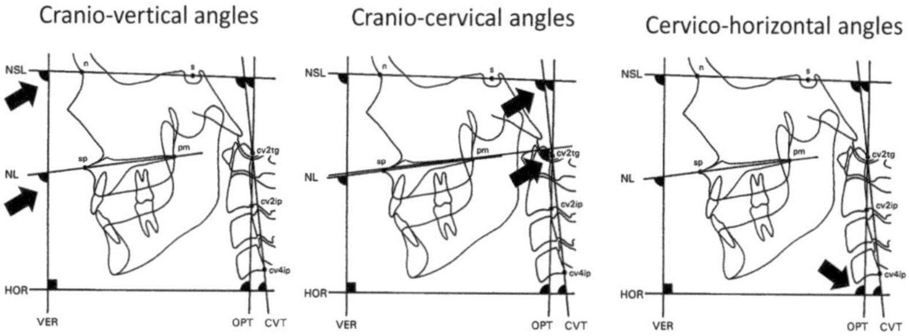

Figure 1. Angles describing the head posture.

Extension of the head means a raised position of the head in relation to the upper spine or true vertical, that is, large cranio-cervical angle (NSL/OPT, NL/OPT, NSL/CVT, NL/CVT) and cranio-vertical angle (NSL/VER, NL/VER), respectively. Forward inclination of the upper spine means a small cervico-horizontal angle (OPT/HOR, CVT/HOR).

2.2. Head posture in OSA patients

In OSA patients, an extended posture of the head in relation to the upper cervical spine in the upright awake position was found to be associated with larger pharyngeal airway dimensions [9, 20–25]. It was especially the lower part of the pharyngeal airway that was increased in relation to an extended head posture. Furthermore, an extended posture of the head has also been demonstrated in men with OSA compared to healthy controls [9, 24] (**Figure 2**).

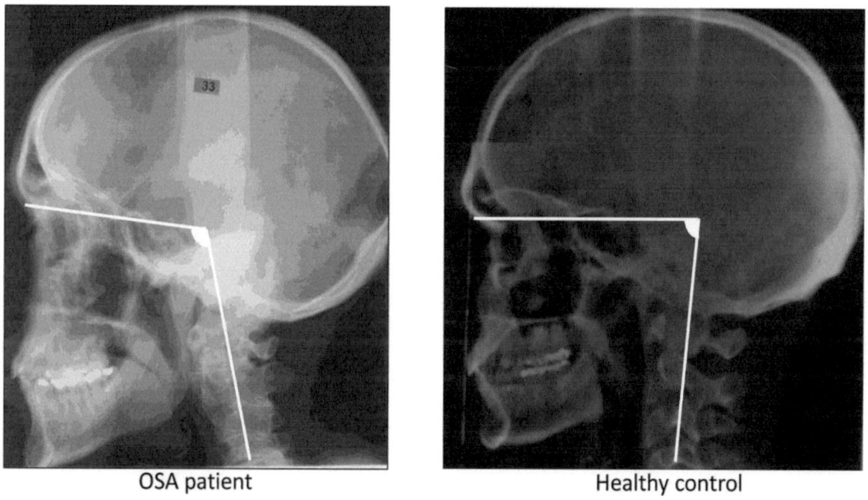

Figure 2. Extended head posture in an OSA patient compared to a healthy control illustrated on lateral cephalograms.

The severity of OSA was also associated with head posture. The more severe OSA, the more extended and forward head posture was observed [20–23]. The extended head posture in OSA patients may be a compensatory physiological postural mechanism that serves to maintain airway adequacy in OSA patients [9, 20–25]. It is suggested that airway obstruction via neuromuscular control triggers an increase in the cranio-cervical angle in order to relieve the obstruction by facilitating oral breathing due to enlargement of the naso-and oropharyngeal airway space [9, 13, 24, 26]. The hypothesis is supported by a study in OSA patients showing that the airway resistance significantly influences the head posture [21]. A decreased airway resistance (less obstructive) was seen in OSA patients with an extended head posture. Thus, an extended head posture in the upright awake position was found in OSA patients. The results were considered to reflect a compensatory physiological postural mechanism that serves to maintain airway adequacy in OSA patients in the awake upright posture.

3. Upper spine morphology in relation to OSA

Until recently, deviations of the upper cervical spine have only been described in relation to craniofacial syndromes and cleft lip and palate. Craniosynostosis syndromes, for example, Pfeiffer's, Crouzon's, and Apert's syndromes, showed deviations such as fusion anomalies [27–31]. Furthermore, deviations of the upper cervical spine morphology were seen in Saethre-Chotzen, Klippel-Feil, Turner, Down syndromes, and patients with hypophosphatemic rickets [32–38]. Also, upper spine morphological deviations have been closely investigated in patients with cleft lip and/or palate [39–44]. Recently, upper spine morphological deviations are also found to be associated with severe malocclusion traits and the craniofacial profile [45–49]. In addition, upper spine morphological deviations are associated with head posture [50–52]. As an association between head posture and OSA and between head posture and upper cervical spine morphology is documented, it seems relevant to focus on the relationship between the morphology of the upper cervical spine and OSA.

3.1. Definition of upper spine morphology

The upper cervical spine morphology can be obtained from conventional two-dimensional (2D) lateral cephalograms or from three-dimensional (3D) cone beam computed tomography (CBCT). One method to describe the upper cervical spine morphology on either lateral cephalograms or on CBCT is by visual assessment of the first five cervical vertebral units as referred to in this chapter. The morphological deviations are divided into two categories "Posterior arch deficiency" and "fusion anomalies" [14, 40, 45] (**Figure 3**):

1. Posterior arch deficiency consisted of *partial cleft*: failure of the posterior part of the neural arch to fuse and *dehiscence*: failure of part of a vertebral unit to develop (**Figure 3**).

2. Fusion anomalies consisted of *fusion*: fusion of one unit with another at the articulation facets, neural arch or transverse processes, *block fusion*: fusion of more than two units at the vertebral bodies, articulation facets, neural arch or transverse processes and *occipitalization*: assimilation either partial or complete of the atlas (C1) with the occipital bone (**Figure 3**).

http://dx.doi.org/10.5772/65436

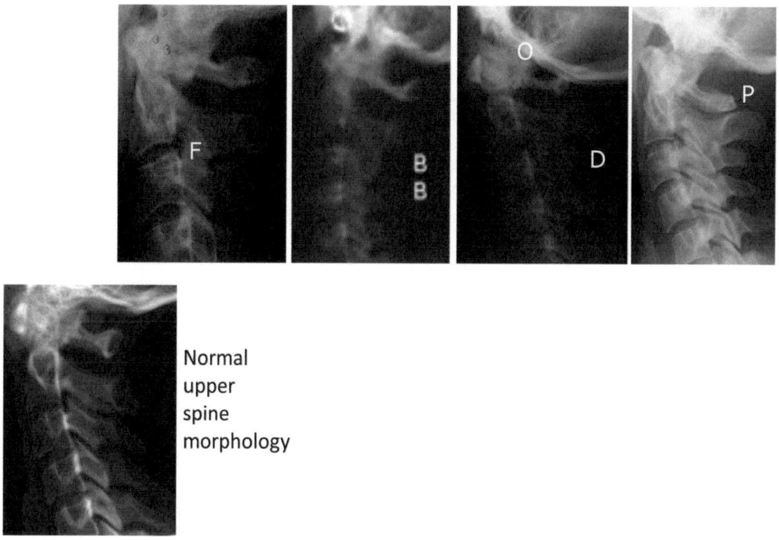

Figure 3. Upper spine morphological deviations and normal upper spine morphology illustrated on lateral cephalograms. P: partial cleft, D: dehiscence, F: fusion, B: block fusion, O: occipitalization.

3.2. Upper spine morphology in OSA patients

Previous studies have shown that morphological deviations in the upper cervical spine evaluated on 2D lateral cephalograms and 3D CBCT occurred significantly more often in OSA patients compared to healthy controls [53, 54]. The morphological deviations occurred in 32–46% as fusion anomalies: fusions either between the second and third vertebrae, between the third and fourth vertebrae, or between the fourth and fifth cervical vertebrae; block fusions: fusions either between the second, third, or fourth vertebrae, between the second, third, fourth, and fifth vertebrae, or between the third, fourth, and fifth vertebrae; occipitali-

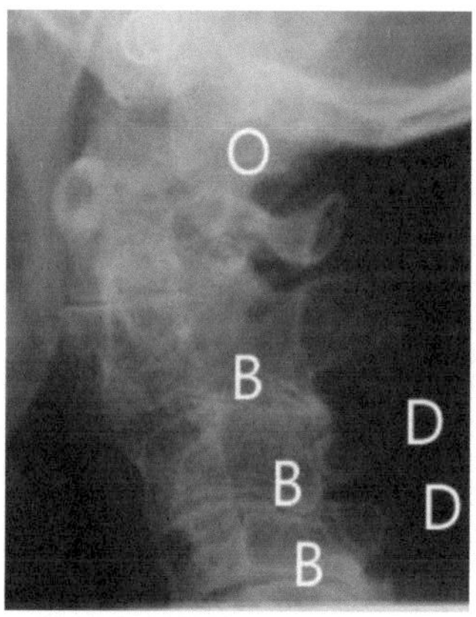

Figure 4. Upper spine morphological deviations in patients with OSA illustrated on lateral cephalograms. O: occipitalization, B: block fusion, D: dehiscence.

zation in combination with fusions, block fusions or as a single deviation. Posterior arch deficiency: partial cleft of the first cervical vertebra or dehiscence of the third cervical vertebra and the fourth cervical vertebra [53, 54] (**Figure 4**). The pattern of morphological deviations in the upper spine seen in OSA patients is more severe and occurred more caudally than seen in healthy subjects and in orthodontic patients with severe malocclusion [45–49]. Occipitalization, block fusion, and dehiscence were the phenotypes, which were characteristic of sleep apnea (**Figure 4**).

It is presumed that the pattern and location of upper cervical spine morphological deviations is connected to different locations of neural crest cell migration along the body axis [55]. Accordingly, it is hypothesized that the level of pharyngeal obstruction in sleep apnea is associated with the caudally/cranially positioned cervical spine deviation. Furthermore, the craniofacial profile of OSA patients with upper spine morphological deviations was significantly different from the craniofacial profile in OSA patients without deviations in the upper spine [56] (**Figure 5**). A long and retrognathic facial profile together with an extended head posture was characteristic of OSA patients with upper spine morphological deviations.

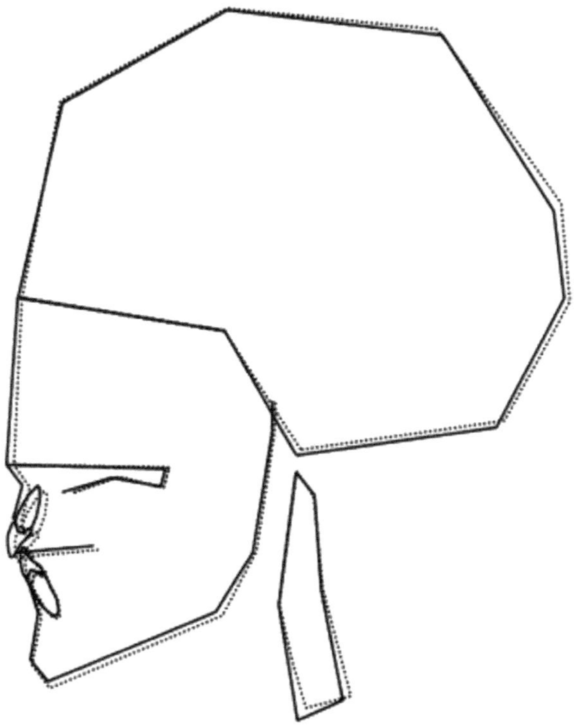

Figure 5. Mean diagrams of OSA patient's craniofacial profile with (dotted line) and without (bold line) upper spine morphological deviations.

The background for the interrelationship between the cervical spine and the craniofacial profile can be traced back to early embryological development of these structures [57]. It has been documented that the development of the body axis is regulated by the notochord [58, 59]. It is also well known that the notochord runs in its full extent from the sacral region to the sella turcica in the posterior part of the cranial base to which the jaws are attached [55]. Different genes act in different segments along the path [60]. A deviation in the development of the notochord may influence the surrounding bone tissue in the spine as well as in the posterior part of the cranial base. On lateral cephalograms and CBCTs, it can be observed that the bone tissues formed around the notochord are the vertebral bodies and the basilar part of the occipital bone (**Figure 6**). The shared origin of the spine and posterior part of the cranial base is the basis for the hypothesis of associations between the spine and the cranial base to which the jaws are attached [60, 61].

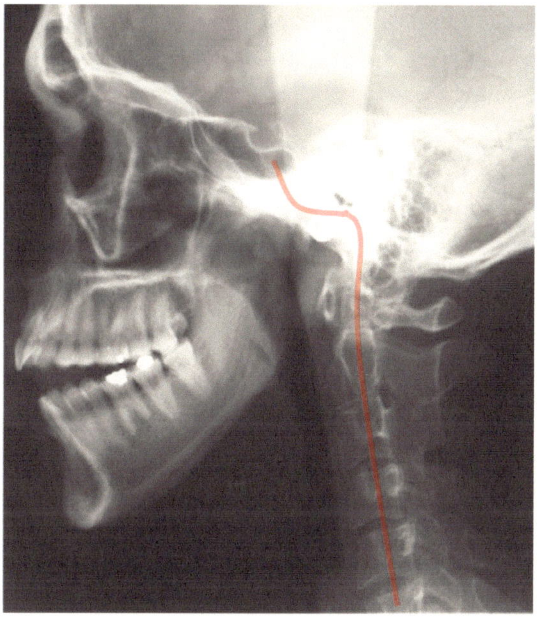

Figure 6. The red line illustrates the extension of the notochord. Note that the notochord disappears in the early embryogenesis before the ossification of the bone tissue.

The findings indicated that morphological deviations of the upper cervical spine may play a role in the phenotypical subdivision and diagnosis of OSA. In addition, OSA patients with morphological deviations in the upper spine may respond poorer to MAD treatment compared to OSA patients without morphological deviations in the upper spine [62]. This finding further supports the role of upper spine morphological deviations in OSA patients. So far, the complex aetiology of OSA is not fully understood and the explanation for the association between upper spine morphological deviations and OSA is still unknown. Thus, the findings indicated that the aetiology in OSA patients with morphological deviations in the upper spine is characterized by other factors or combinations of different factors than in OSA patients without upper spine morphological deviations and that upper spine morphological deviations therefore may influence the MAD treatment outcome in OSA patient [53, 54, 56, 62].

4. Conclusion

When head position and upper cervical spine morphological deviations are evaluated on 2D lateral cephalograms and 3D CBCTs taken in the standardized upright position of the head determined by the subjects' own postural control system, the following is concluded: on average, an extended posture of the head and a significantly larger occurrence of upper spine morphological deviations were seen in patients with OSA. The craniofacial profile of OSA patients with upper cervical spine morphological deviations differed significantly from the craniofacial profile of other OSA patients without morphological deviations in the upper spine. OSA patients with morphological deviations in the upper spine may respond poorer to MAD treatment compared to OSA patients without morphological deviations in the upper spine. The findings indicated that head posture and morphological deviations of the upper cervical spine play a role in the phenotypical subdivision and diagnosis of OSA and thereby for the treatment outcome.

Author details

Liselotte Sonnesen

Address all correspondence to: alson@sund.ku.dk

Department of Odontology, Faculty of Medical Health and Sciences, Copenhagen University, Copenhagen, Denmark

References

[1] Prisant LM, Dillard TA, Blanchard AR. Obstructive sleep apnea syndrome. J Clin Hypertens (Greenwich). 2006;8:746–750.

[2] Wolkove N, Elkholy O, Baltzan M, Palayew M. Sleep and aging: 1. Sleep disorders commonly found in older people. CMAJ. 2007;176:1299–1304.

[3] Guilleminault C, Tilkian A, Dement WC. The sleep apnea syndromes. Annu Rev Med. 1976;27:465–484.

[4] Balachandran JS, Patel SR. In the clinic. Obstructive sleep apnea. Ann Intern Med. 2014;161:ITC1.

[5] Ngiam J, Balasubramaniam R, Darendeliler MA, Cheng AT, Waters K, Sullivan CE. Clinical guidelines for oral appliance therapy in the treatment of snoring and obstructive sleep apnea. Aust Dent J. 2013;58:408–419.

[6] Epstein LJ Kristo, D, Strollo Jr., PJ, Friedman N. Clinical guideline for the evaluation, management and long-term care of obstructive sleep apnea in adults. J Clin Sleep Med. 2009;5:263–276.

[7] Jordan AS, McSharry DG, Malhotra A. Adult obstructive sleep apnoea. Lancet. 2014;383:736–747.

[8] Neelapu BC, Kharbanda OP, Sardana HK, Balachandran R, Sardana V, Kapoor P, Gupta A, Vasamsetti S. Craniofacial and upper airway morphology in adult obstructive sleep apnea patients: a systematic review and meta-analysis of cephalometric studies. Sleep Med Rev. 2016.DOI: 10.1016/j.smrv.2016.01.007.

[9] Solow B, Skov S, Ovesen J, Norup PW, Wildschiødtz G. Airway dimensions and head posture in obstructive sleep apnoea. Eur J Orthod. 1996;18(6):571–579.

[10] Anegawa E, Tsuyama H, Kusukawa J. Lateral cephalometric analysis of the pharyngeal airway space affected by headposture. Int J Oral Maxillofac Surg. 2008;37:805–809.

[11] Muto T, Takeda S, Kanazawa M, Yamazaki A, Fujiwara Y, Mizoguchi I. The effect of head posture on the pharyngeal airway space (PAS). Int J Oral Maxillofac Surg. 2002;31:579–583.

[12] Hellsing E. Changes in the pharyngeal airway in relation to extension of the head. Eur J Orthod. 1989;11(4):359–365.

[13] Solow B, Sandham A. Cranio-cervical posture: a factor in the development and function of the dentofacial structures. Eur J Orthod. 2002;24(5):447–456.

[14] Sonnesen L. Head posture and upper spine morphology in relation to the craniofacial profile and orofacial function. In: Curran SA, editor. Posture: Types, Exercises and Health Effects. Nova Science Publishers, Inc. USA.; 2014. Chapter 3, p. 43–55.

[15] Moorrees CF. Natural head position-a revival. Am J Orthod Dentofacial Orthop. 1994;105(5):512–513.

[16] Molhave A. A biostatic investigation. The standing posture of man theoretically and statometrically illustrated. Acta Orthop Scand. 1960;29:291–300.

[17] Solow B, Tallgren A. Natural head position in standing subjects. Acta Odont Scand. 1971;29:591–607.

[18] Solow B, Tallgren A. Craniocervical posture in relation to skeletal and dentoalveolar morphology. Trans Eur Orthodon Soc. 1975;231–235.

[19] Solow B, Tallgren A. Head posture and craniofacial morphology. Am J Phys Anthropol. 1976;44:417–435.

[20] Tong M, Sakakibara H, Xia X, Suetsugu S. Compensatory head posture changes in patients with obstructive sleep apnea. J Tongji Med Univ. 2000;20(1):66–69.

[21] Choi JK, Goldman M, Koyal S, Clark G. Effect of jaw and head position on airway resistance in obstructive sleep apnea. Sleep Breath. 2000;4(4):163–168.

[22] Tangugsorn V, Krogstad O, Espeland L, Lyberg T. Obstructive sleep apnea (OSA): a cephalometric analysis of severe and non-severe OSA patients. Part I: multiple comparison of cephalometric variables. Int J Adult Orthodon Orthognath Surg. 2000;15(2): 139–152.

[23] Ozbek MM, Miyamoto K, Lowe AA, Fleetham JA. Natural head posture, upper airway morphology and obstructive sleep apnoea severity in adults. Eur J Orthod. 1998;20(2): 133–143.

[24] Solow B, Ovesen J, Nielsen PW, Wildschiødtz G, Tallgren A. Head posture in obstructive sleep apnoea. Eur J Orthod. 1993;15(2):107–114.

[25] Tangugsorn V, Skatvedt O, Krogstad O, Lyberg T. Obstructive sleep apnoea: a cephalometric study. Part I. Cervico-craniofacial skeletal morphology. Eur J Orthod. 1995;17(1):45–56.

[26] Solow B, Kreiborg S. Soft-tissue stretching: a possible control factor in craniofacial morphogenesis. Scand J Dent Res. 1977;85:505–507.

[27] Hemmer KM, McAlister WH, Marsh JL. Cervical spine anomalies in the craniosynostosis syndromes. Cleft Palate J. 1987;24(4):328–333.

[28] Kreiborg S, Barr Jr M, Cohen Jr MM. Cervical spine in the Apert syndrome. Am J Med Genet. 1992; 43(4):704–708.

[29] Anderson PJ, Hall CM, Evans RD, Jones BM, Harkness W, Hayvard RD. The cervical spine in Pfeiffer's syndrome. J Craniofac Surg. 1996;7(4):275–279.

[30] Anderson PJ, Hall C, Evans RD, Jones BM, Harkness WJ, Hayward RD. The cervical spine in Crouzon syndrome. Spine. 1997;22(4):402–405.

[31] Thompson DNP, Slaney SF, Hall CM, Shaw D, Jones BM, Hayward RD. Congenital cervical spinal fusion: a study in Apert syndrome. Pediatr Neurosurg. 1996;25(1):22–27.

[32] Anderson PJ, Hall CM, Evans RD, Hayward RD, Harkness WJ, Jones BM. The cervical spine in Saethre-Chotzen syndrome. Cleft Palate Craniofac J. 1997;34(1):79–82.

[33] Frost M, Huffer WE, Sze CI, Badesch D, Cajade-Law AG, Kleinschmidt-Demasters BK. Cervical spine abnormalities in Down syndrome. Clin Neuropathol. 1999;18(5); 250–259.

[34] Trusen A, Beissert M, Collmann H, Darge K. The pattern of skeletal anomalies in the cervical spine, hands and feet in patients with Saethre-Chotzen syndrome and Muenke type mutation. Pediatr Radiol. 2003;33(3):168–172.

[35] Samartzis D, Herman J, Lubicky JP, Shen FH. Classification of congenitally fused cervical patterns in Klippel-Feil patients: epidemiology and role in the development of

cervical spine-related symptoms. Spine. 2006;31(21):E798–E804. DOI:10.1097/01.brs. 0000239222.36505.46

[36] Shen FH, Samartzis D, Herman, Lubicky JP. Radiographic assessment of segmental motion at the atlantoaxial junction in the Klippel-Feil patient. Spine. 2006; 31(2):171–177.

[37] Gjørup H, Sonnesen L, Beck-Nielsen SS, Haubek D. Upper spine morphology in hypophosphatemic rickets and healthy controls: a radiographic study. Eur J Orthod. 2014;36(2):217–225.

[38] Michelsen T, Brusgaard P, Sonnesen L. Klippel-Feil: a syndrome in the occipital-cervical spine field and its dentofacial manifestations. World J Stomatol. 2015;20(2):81–86.

[39] Ross RB, Lindsay WK. The cervical vertebrae as a factor in etiology of cleft palate. Cleft Palate J. 1965;36:273–281.

[40] Sandham A. Cervical vertebral anomalies in cleft lip and palate. Cleft Palate J. 1986;23(3):206–214.

[41] Horswell BB. The incidence and relationship of cervical spine anomalies in patients with cleft lip and/or palate. J Oral Maxillofac Surg. 1991;49(7):693–697.

[42] Hoenig JF, Schoener WF. Radiological survey of the cervical spine in cleft lip and palate. Dentomaxillofac Radiol.1992;21(1):36–39.

[43] Ugar DA, Semb G. The prevalence of anomalies of the upper cervical vertebrae in subjects with cleft lip, cleft palate, or both. Cleft Palate Craniofac J. 2001;38(5):498–503.

[44] Rajion ZA, Townsend GC, Netherway DJ, et al. A threedimensional computed tomographic analysis of the cervical spine in unoperated infants with cleft lip and palate. Cleft Palate Craniofac J. 2006;43(5):513–518.

[45] Sonnesen L. Associations between the cervical vertebral column and craniofacial morphology. Int J Dent. 2010;2010:295728. DOI: 10.1155/2010/295728.

[46] Sonnesen L, Kjaer I. Cervical column morphology in patients with skeletal Class III malocclusion and mandibular overjet. Am J Orthod Dentofacial Orthop. 2007;132(4): 427.e7–12. DOI:10.1016/j.ajodo.2007.01.019

[47] Sonnesenn L, Kjaer I. Cervical vertebral body fusions in patients with skeletal deep bite. Eur J Orthod. 2007;29(5):464–470.

[48] Sonnesen L, Kjaer I. Anomalies of the cervical vertebrae in patients with skeletal Class II malocclusion and horizontal maxillary overjet. Am J Orthod Dentofacial Orthop. 2008;133(2):188.e15–20. DOI: 10.1016/j.ajodo.2007.07.018.

[49] Sonnesen L, Kjaer I. Cervical column morphology in patients with skeletal open bite. Orthod Craniofacial Res. 2008;11(1):17–23.

[50] Sonnesen L, Pedersen CE, Kjær I. Cervical column morphology related to head posture, cranial base angle, and condylar malformation. Eur J Orthod. 2007;29(4):398–403.

[51] Arntsen T, Sonnesen L. Cervical vertebral column morphology related to craniofacial morphology and head posture in preorthodontic children with Class II malocclusion and horizontal maxillary overjet. Am J Orthod Dentofacial Orthop. 2011;140(1):e1–7.

[52] Kim P, Sarauw MT, Sonnesen L. Cervical vertebral column morphology and head posture in preorthodontic patients with anterior open bite. Am J Orthod Dentofacial Orthop. 2014;145(3):359–366.

[53] Sonnesen L, Petri N, Kjaer I, Svanholt P. Cervical column morphology in adult patients with obstructive sleep apnoea. Eur J Orthod. 2008;30:521–526.

[54] Sonnesen L, Jensen KE, Petersson AR, Petri N, Berg S, Svanholt P. Cervical vertebral column morphology in patients with obstructive sleep apnoea assessed using lateral cephalograms and cone beam CT. A comparative study. Dentomaxillofac Radiol. 2013; 42:20130060. DOI: 10.1259/dmfr.20130060 DOI:10.1259%2Fdmfr.20130060 #pmc_ext.

[55] Kjaer I. Neuroosteology. Crit Rev Oral Biol Med. 1999;9:224–244.

[56] Svanholt P, Petri N, Wildschiødtz G, Sonnesen L, Kjaer I. Associations between craniofacial morphology, head posture, and cervical vertebral body fusions in men with sleep apnoea. Am J Orthod Dentofac Orthop. 2009;135:702.e1–9.

[57] Kjaer I. Human prenatal craniofacial development related to brain development under normal and pathological conditions. Acta Odontol Scand. 1995;53:135–143.

[58] Kjaer I, Kjær TW, Græm N. Ossification sequence of occipital bone and vertebrae in human fetuses. J Craniofac Genet Dev Biol. 1993;13:83–88.

[59] Nolting D, Hansen BF, Keeling J, Kjaer I. Prenatal development of the human vertebral corpora in different segments of the spine. Spine. 1998;23:2265–2271.

[60] Sonnesen L, Nolting D, Kjaer KW, Kjaer I. Association between the development of the body axis and the craniofacial skeleton studied by immunohistochemical analyses using collagen II, Pax9, Pax1, and Noggin antibodies. Spine (Phila Pa 1976). 2008;33(15): 1622–6.

[61] Sonnesen L, Nolting D, Engel U, Kjaer I. Cervical vertebrae, cranial base, and mandibular retrognathia in human triploid fetuses. Am J Med Genet A. 2009;149A(2):177–187.

[62] Svanholt P, Petri N, Wildschiødtz G, Sonnesen L. Influence of craniofacial and upper spine morphology on mandibular advancement device treatment outcome in patients with obstructive sleep apnoea: a pilot study. Eur J Orthod. 2015;37:391–397.